Basics of
Electrotherapy

Basics of Electrotherapy

Subhash Khatri

BPh.T (Nagpur), MPT Ortho (Kottayam)
Associate Professor and Head
Department of Physiotherapy
Jawaharlal Nehru Medical College
Belgaum

JAYPEE BROTHERS
MEDICAL PUBLISHERS (P) LTD.
New Delhi

Published by

Jitendar P Vij
Jaypee Brothers Medical Publishers (P) Ltd
EMCA House, 23/23B Ansari Road, Daryaganj
New Delhi 110 002, India
Phones: 23272143, 23272703, 23282021, 23245672, 23245683
Fax: 011-23276490   e-mail: jpmedpub@del2.vsnl.net.in
Visit our website: http://www.jpbros.20m.com

Branches

- 202 Batavia Chambers, 8 Kumara Kruppa Road, Kumara Park East,
  Bangalore 560 001, Phones: 2285971, 2382956 Tele Fax: 2281761
  e-mail: jaypeebc@bgl.vsnl.net.in

- 282 IIIrd Floor, Khaleel Shirazi Estate, Fountain Plaza
  Pantheon Road, **Chennai** 600 008, Phone: 28262665 Fax: 28262331
  e-mail: jpmedpub@md3.vsnl.net.in

- 4-2-1067/1-3, Ist Floor, Balaji Building, Ramkote
  Cross Road, **Hyderabad** 500 095, Phones: 55610020, 24758498
  Fax: 24758499   e-mail: jpmedpub@rediffmail.com

- 1A Indian Mirror Street, Wellington Square
  Kolkata 700 013, Phone: 22451926 Fax: 22456075
  e-mail: jpbcal@cal.vsnl.net.in

- 106 Amit Industrial Estate, 61 Dr SS Rao Road, Near MGM Hospital
  Parel, **Mumbai** 400 012 , Phones: 24124863, 24104532 Fax: 24160828
  e-mail: jpmedpub@bom7.vsnl.net.in

Basics of Electrotherapy

First Edition: **2003**

Publishing Director: RK Yadav

ISBN 81-8061-171-X

Typeset at   JPBMP typesetting unit
Printed at   Gopsons Papers Ltd., A-14, Sector 60,Noida

*In loving memory of my father Maniklal
Khatri who raised me, guided me and
believed in me no matter what. I could
not have asked for a better teacher and
mentor than my father.*

to
my daughter 'Trishala'

Preface

Day today we come across various physical forces such as warming rays of sun, light of moon, force of gravity, movement of our body, our ability to move from one place to another, our ability to move an object from one place to another, movement and flow of cold and hot water, electrical changes, magnetism and so on. Almost all these things around us form the part of nature's inexhaustible and powerful array of forces. The same physical forces, harnessed and properly directed are of great value in promoting the healing. They can relieve pain, increase circulation, speed up repair and healing of injured body part, improve body mechanics, metabolism, inhibit growth of germs, restore disturbed function, cure the diseased status of body, restore homeostasis, improve health and so on. This could be the basis of physical medicine. It appears that the evolution of Physical Medicine or Physiotherapy has occurred gradually but the physical agents in some or the other form, which are used for the treatment purpose, are reasonably old, may be as old as matter itself.

Electrotherapy is an essential and basic subject for undergraduate and postgraduate physiotherapy students. There are enough and more books available on this subject by western authors. But personally I feel that there are very few books available on this subject by Indian authors who can understand their needs in better way. So a need was felt to bring out a book, which will comprehensively cover Electrotherapy. The purpose of this book is to provide a foundation of knowledge for the management of most of the type of the patients with the

Electrotherapeutic modalities. I have tried to write the chapters in such a way that as if I was sitting in front of you and trying to explain the matter and hence you may feel as if you were reading my lecture notes. I have also included my memory tricks for remembering the subject matter; you may use them if it works for you. Although the book is primarily written for physiotherapeutic professionals, much of the information in this book may be useful for other clinicians who are actively involved in the management of various patients.

Medical and Physiotherapy knowledge is constantly changing. As new information becomes available, changes in treatment procedures, equipment and the use of these equipments in clinical situations become necessary. The author has as far as possible taken care to ensure that information given in this book is accurate and up-to-date. However, readers are strongly advised to confirm the information. A large number of references and suggested readings have been included at the end. This will help more interested readers to conveniently look for extra material on the subject of their interest.

I have received valuable assistance from various people in the preparation of this book, *Basics of Electrotherapy*. I would like to thank all of them for their suggestions and help. I am particularly thankful to my students and colleagues who inspired me and provided important feedback. I am grateful to my brothers Mohanlal Khatri, Dr Jeevan Khatri and Sanjay kumar Khatri for their constant encouragement and support in various ways. For the help in the typing and correction of the manuscript I am indebted to my wife Mrs Sejal Khatri and my clinical assistant Dr Poonam Bagi.

The publisher M/s Jaypee Brothers Medical Publishers (P) Ltd, New Delhi bestowed upon this work with their highly painstaking efforts in the examination of this text, its editing and printing. The author hereby thankfully acknowledges all of this assistance. I am thankful to Principal Dr VD Patil, JN Medical College, Belgaum for kind permission to publish this book.

I would appreciate your comments about this book. I have included my personal thought and comments and they should be taken as just guidelines.

Subhash Khatri

Contents

Contents

What is Electrotherapy?

DEFINITION AND AREAS OF STUDY

Electrotherapy generally includes various forms of therapeutic applications using electricity as the primary source of energy. In order to have comprehensive idea, first let's try to understand the meaning of the word therapy. The dictionary meaning of the word therapy is non-surgical treatment approach. Electro means electrical current or electricity or electrical means. Hence, one can say that electrotherapy is a non-surgical treatment approach characterized by the treatment of various diseases and disorders with the help of electricity or electrical means. Alternatively one can put it this way; 'Electrotherapy is a branch of physiotherapy characterized by the treatment of various diseases and disorders with the help of electricity or electrical means'. In my view, it is one of the essential basic subjects for physiotherapy students. The scope or outline of electrotherapy can be understood with the help of following diagram.

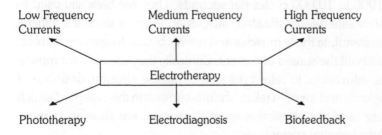

Fig. 1.1: Areas of study in electrotherapy

If you see the figure 1.1 then you might have noticed that there are two common words, one is frequency and the second is current. Current is nothing but the flow of electrons. Frequency is the number of occurrence of any event per unit time. If you take five cups of coffee per day then I may say that your frequency of coffee intake is five cups per day. Similarly if you are a smoker and smoke three cigarettes per day then the frequency of your smoking is three cigarettes per day. With this kind of analogy let's try to understand the use of word frequency in electrotherapy. In electrotherapy, we use the currents whose impulses commence and cease at regular interval. The number of times these impulses comes in a particular unit time (second) is regarded as frequency. Usually it is expressed in cycles per second or hertz, kilohertz, megahertz, etc.

Low frequency currents Low frequency currents are therapeutically used currents whose frequency is in the range of 0 to 100 cycles per second. The primary use of low frequency current is the stimulation of nerve and muscle. Various current in this category which are used for the physiotherapeutic treatments are direct current, interrupted direct current, sinusoidal current, diadynamic current, high voltage pulsed galvanic current, micro amperage electrical nerve stimulation, transcutaneous electrical nerve stimulation, etc.

Medium frequency currents Medium frequency currents are therapeutically used currents whose frequency is in the range of 1000 to 10,000 cycles per seconds. They are basically used to stimulate deeply situated muscles and nerves since it's difficult to stimulate these muscles and nerves by low frequency currents without the spread of current. Clinically they are used for muscle re-education, to retard the rate of muscle atrophy, drainage of edema and for pain relief. Various currents in this category, which are used for physiotherapeutic purpose, are Russian current, Interferential current, etc.

High frequency currents   High frequency currents are therapeutically used currents whose frequency is more than 10,000 cycles per seconds. High frequency currents are used for their ability to produce the deep heat inside the tissues. Various electrotherapeutic modalities, which work on this type of currents, are short wave diathermy, long wave diathermy, therapeutic ultrasound, and microwave diathermy.

Phototherapy   Phototherapy refers to the treatment of various diseases and disorders with the help of light. The primary effect of these phototherapeutic modalities is pain relief by heat and acceleration of healing through elevation of temperature, counterirritation and photochemical effects. Various modalities such as infrared rays, ultraviolet rays and laser comes under this category.

Electrodiagnosis   Electrical currents can also be used for the diagnostic purpose. Electrodiagnosis means the detection of the diseases and disorders by the use of electrotherapeutic currents or electromyography. We can use currents like interrupted direct current and perform various electrodiagnostic tests such as rheobase, chronaxie, strength duration curve, pulse ratio, myasthenic reaction, galvanic tetanic ratio, nerve conduction test, nerve distribution test, faradic galvanic test, etc. Electromyography is the study of electrical activity of the muscle by means of surface electrodes placed over the skin or needle electrodes inserted in the muscle itself. By electromyography we can study motor unit potential, motor nerve conduction velocity, sensory nerve conduction velocity, etc.

Biofeedback   Biofeedback is the process of furnishing the information to an individual about the body function so as to get some voluntary control over it. Some biofeedback devices are related to electrotherapy and hence, they can be included under electrotherapy for example EMG biofeedback. However, one should remember that there are lot many biofeedback devices which works on mechanical principles.

CLASSIFICATION OF CURRENTS

Therapeutic currents can be classified on the basis of direction, frequency, voltage, amperage and biophysical effects in different ways.

On the basis of direction   On the basis of the direction of the flow, therapeutic currents can be classified as alternating and unidirectional currents. Unidirectional currents are those that flow in one direction only for example direct current and interrupted direct current. Alternating currents flow in both the directions. Examples of this type of currents are sinusoidal current and interferential currents.

On the basis of frequency   On the basis of the frequency therapeutic currents can be classified as low frequency, medium frequency and high frequency currents. Examples and more about these currents are mentioned earlier.

On the basis of voltage   On this basis, therapeutic currents are classified as low voltage and high voltage currents. Low voltage currents are with a voltage of less than 100 volts for example low frequency currents. High voltage currents are of several hundred volts for example high frequency currents.

On the basis of amperage   On the basis of amperage the currents are divided into two types such as low amperage and high amperage currents. Low amperage currents area those currents whose amperage ranges from 1 to 30 milliampears and are same as that of low voltage currents. High amperage currents have amperage from 500 to 2000 milliampears and are usually of high tension.

On the basis of biophysical effects   On this basis currents can be divided into two types such as currents causing ionic changes and currents causing thermal changes.

I always get surprised to see a chapter on cold therapy in electrotherapy textbooks and similarly chapters on paraffin wax bath, hot pack, contrast bath, etc. One may think that it is not the part of electrotherapy but traditionally cold is described along with heat and hence mostly we find that cold therapy and other things such as paraffin wax bath, hot pack, contrast bath, fluidotherapy, etc. are often described in electrotherapy textbooks. However, personally I like the authors who put the title of their textbook as physical agents since it avoids the dilemma of what can be included in electrotherapy. One should be aware of the fact that all physiotherapy modalities which work on electricity may not be necessarily called as electrotherapeutic modalities. I always remember one of the professor asking this question to undergraduate students, is traction an electrotherapy modality? Of course the answer is no. But few students may get confused and may say yes. We have continuous passive motion devices, intermittent compression devices and traction machines, which may work on electricity but should not be ideally called as electrotherapy modalities!

Students of physical therapy must appreciate that any form of physical energy applied to the body exert significant primary as well as secondary physiological effects. There is a need to accurately measure the dosages in the application of all physical agents just as in the use of medication, there is a therapeutic range required to achieve the desired effects. Too low an intensity may not produce any physiological changes and too high a dose may produce serious detrimental consequences. Also as in medication, there is need to determine when to discontinue the use of these electrotherapeutic procedures. They cannot be utilized indiscriminately by using it almost indefinitely in patients who may not further benefit from its continued use. However, we should keep in mind that even if we use too many sophisticated or complicated electrotherapy machines in treating the patients, they just form the part of total physiotherapy management and we should not forget other things, at least we should not forget the human touch what we could always offer to our patients through manual therapy.

SUMMARY

Various areas of study in electrotherapy are low frequency currents, medium frequency currents, high frequency currents, phototherapy, electrodiagnosis and biofeedback. Low frequency currents are used for stimulation of muscles and nerves. Medium frequency currents are used for re-education of deeply situated muscles, pain relief and for drainage of edema. High frequency currents are used for the production of deep heat inside the tissues. Phototherapy is used for pain relief and acceleration of healing. Electrodiagnosis helps in the study of electrical reactions of muscles and nerves for the diagnostic purpose.

chapter two

History of Electrotherapy

Well, you must have got wondered to see a chapter on history of electrotherapy in this book. I always tell my students about the importance of knowing the history. I feel that one's knowledge is always incomplete without knowing the history of that subject. The knowledge of the history helps in knowing the subject in depth and philosophically it is also said that when one is aware of the history then he won't repeat the same mistake done by others in the past.

Here is the abstract form of historical aspects of electrotherapy. In 1646, Sir Thomas Browne, physician used the word Electricity for the first time. Aetius, a Greek physician had prescribed the shocks of Torpedo, an electric fish for the treatment of gout. By1780, Luigi Galvani a professor of the anatomy at the faculty of Bologna, first observed the quick twitching of the muscle produced by the electricity in a nerve muscle preparation of the frog's leg. History records that famous French physicist Abbe Nollet administered the shock from Leyden jar to 180 royal guards simultaneously in presence of the King. Johann Gottlob Kruger, professor of Medicine at Halle, Germany gave a series of lectures to medical students in 1743 entitled thoughts about the electricity. These were published in 1744 enlarged by notes and reprinted the following year. It was the first book on medical electricity, although subsequent book written by his pupil Christian Gottlieb Kratzenstein and published in 1745 was the first to use medical electricity in its title.

Richard Lovett in England treated many persons with static shocks and published a treatise in 1756 describing the numerous conditions for which electrotherapy was to be recommended. John Wesley, the religious leader became interested in his work and published his own experiences on the subject in 1759 in the book titled the Desideratum. Bertholon described his techniques with its role in the cure of eight paralytics. In 1768 an electrotherapy instrument was installed at Middlesex hospital in London. The electrical department established at Guys hospital in London is now historically recognized as the first hospital physical therapy department. Electrotherapy received another boost when the renowned physician S. Weir Mitchell, endorsed exercises of muscles by faradic stimulation. Surprisingly, I came to know that once upon a time Electrotherapy was supposed to be the part of radiology through professor Nayak, honorary professor of radiology at JN Medical College, Belgaum. Of course later on I got the similar reference from one of the textbook on this matter by a Philippine based author.

It is interesting to note that due to many similarities, the development of radiology and electrotherapy paralleled each other. Electrical machines were placed along side X-ray machines in hospitals. By 1919, physiotherapy became an adjunct of radiology in the years prior to and immediately after World War II.

Muscle Nerve Stimulation

In 1780 professor Luigi Galvani, professor of anatomy at the faculty of Boulogne first observed the twitching of frog's leg muscles by electricity. Twenty years later Volta proved that this was due to sudden make of the current flow in an electric cell. In 1831 Faraday discovered induction or faradic coil. The man probably did the most to place electrotherapy on scientific level clinically was Guillaume Benjamin Amand Duchenne of

Boulogne who in 1855 described its application for electrical stimulation of muscles and recommended the localized application of faradic current in the treatment of muscle atrophy. Reamak first demonstrated the motor points for accurate electrical testing of muscles. Dubois Reymond in 1849 formulated the law of electrical muscle and nerve stimulation and first used the induction coil for muscle stimulation. Leduc introduced an interrupted direct current. In 1934 Morris reasoned out that denervated muscle will not contract unless the stimulus last for about 100 milliseconds.

Iontophoresis

The idea of driving the drugs in the body through the skin by means of electric current was advanced by Private in 1747. For many years the iodide remained the favorite for the trial introduction, as its recovery through the urine was conclusive. In 1888, Erb recovered electrically driven iodide from the saliva and urine of the patient. In the same year Arrhenius published his thesis on electrolytic dissociation and the process had been incorrectly termed ionization since then up until the end of second World War. During the last decade of the 19th century Ensch scooped a weal out of a potato and filled it with a solution of potassium iodide. He then applied wires into each side of the potato and passed the current through it. Starch in the potato turned blue at the positive pole. The experiment was popularized by Schazki of Russia and was possibly the most quoted work on the new start of therapeutic ion transfer. Stephan Leduc of the France proposed a unit of the dosage as one milliampere per square centimeter of electrode surface. In addition to this hydroelectric baths were first advocated by Sere.

High Frequency Currents

Historically treatment with the high frequency current was also called as electropyrexia, thermopenetration, transthermy, heating through, etc. In 1842 American physicist Joseph Henry observed that the discharges from the Leyden jar condensor were of oscillating character. By 1892 Arsene D'Arsonval of Paris developed an apparatus capable of producing high frequency current of several thousand oscillations per second and was the first person to study effect of high frequency current on human. In 1891 Nicola Tesla in United States observed the heating action of high frequency current. In 1899 Von Zeyneck published a paper in which briefly mentioned about 'Durch warming' or 'Heating through' of his fingertips when an alternating current passed through them. In 1907 Zyneck of Germany with Austrians Preyss and Berend used high frequency current on animals. They also treated gonorrheal arthritis with an apparatus producing damped oscillations and called this method of treating as thermopenetration. In 1908 Nagel Schmidt in Berlin made experiments independently and named his method as transthermy later changing it to diathermy. Thus Nagel Schmidt was the first person to coin the word diathermy. He also demonstrated a more powerful form of it, which left no doubt about the deep heating effects of high frequency current. Diathermy reached its greatest popularity in 1929 when the King of England, who had worsened on ultraviolet ray treatment, was improved by diathermy. Microwave diathermy was the sequence of the development of radar during second World War. In 1928 AW Hull invented the magnetron. Hallman of Germany and his associates did the first study on the biological effects of continuously emitted microwaves. By 1946 Frank H Krusen and his coworkers reported first clinical microwave heating. By the end of the eighteenth century Spallanzani recognized the existence of sound inaudible to human ear. Pierre Currie found one of the best methods of producing ultrasound waves with the quartz crystal. By 1910, Langevin of France produced the first piezoelectric generator for practical use of ultrasound.

Phototherapy

Until seventeenth century, people had difficulty in describing the colours. Some thought that when light passed through a red glass it emerged as red as it was dyed by the glass. In 1801 Johann Wilhelm Ritter called the invisible rays beyond the violet as ultravioletten. At that time the measurement of the wavelength had not yet been fully developed and Ritter used the word ultra, which means beyond. Since ultraviolet rays are actually below, it would have been more accurate to use the term infraviolet. By remarkable coincidence a similar error was done by Herschel the year before in labeling the red rays as infrared. In 1868 Anders Jons Angstrom, Swedish physicist mapped out the wavelength of invisible spectrum and published his results. Then the old unit of the wavelength of measurement was named in his honour as Angstrom unit. At the beginning of twentieth century, the work of Bernhard and Rollier focused on the use of ultraviolet rays in the treatment of extra pulmonary tuberculosis. By 1910, electrically produced ultraviolet generator became commercially available. With the popularity of ultraviolet rays it was easier for the manufacturers to convert the ultraviolet lamps to infrared burners and soon they started promoting them as superior to ultraviolet lamps. However, JH Kellog gave the impetus for the use of infrared rays. In 1981 Kellog built a device similar to heat cradle or baker with 40 lamps of 20 candlepower.

Medical Use of Electricity

After Galvani's experiments Humboldt then proposed the question; can galvanism recall a person to his life who has just died? This question obviously raised snickers among many physicians then but it is of interest to note that a century and half later it is used for just that purpose. Today electric defibrillators are used in cardiac arrest and electric implants are used for the stimulation of phrenic nerve in diaphragmatic paralysis as those seen in poliomyelitis.

SUMMARY

In 1646, Sir Thomas Browne, physician used the word electricity for the first time. Aetius, a Greek physician has prescribed the shocks of Torpedo, an electric fish for the treatment of gout. Johann Gottlob Kruger, professor of Medicine at Halle, Germany published the first book on medical electricity, although subsequent book written by his pupil Christian Gottlieb Kratznstein and published in 1745 was the first to use medical electricity in its title. In 1768 an electrotherapy instrument was installed at Middlesex hospital in London. Electrotherapy received another boost when the renowned physician S. Weir Mitchell, endorsed exercises of muscles by faradic stimulation. Electrical machines were placed along side X-ray machines in hospitals!

chapter three

Muscle Nerve Stimulating Currents

As I mentioned in the second chapter, muscle nerve stimulating currents are used primarily for muscle re-education, pain relief and to delay atrophy and wasting of muscles. In this chapter I have included direct current, faradic current, interrupted direct current, TENS, interferential current, sinusoidal current, diadynamic current, high voltage pulsed galvanic current and HVPG.

DIRECT CURRENT

Direct current is unidirectional continuous current. It is also termed as Galvanic current or plane Galvanic current as an honour to professor Luigi Galvani, professor of anatomy who stimulated muscles and nerves of frog with direct current in 1786. It is also called as constant current, as the current passes continuously in same direction. Direct current is mainly used for iontophoresis, anodal galvanism, cathodal galvanism and for the acceleration of healing.

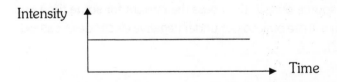

Fig. 3.1: Schematic representation of direct current

Production

Direct current can be obtained from dry batteries as well as from household alternating current. From dry batteries: Here dry batteries or cells are connected in series and a variable resistance controls output. Voltmeter or ammeter can be added to this so as to measure the intensity or output. From alternating current source: Here AC voltage is reduced with the help of a step down transformer. It is rectified and smoothened to get direct current. Output is controlled via variable resistance and can be measured by voltmeter.

Polarity

Polarity is generally marked with direct current source by colour codes for example, red for positive and black for negative. It may be tested with two simple experiments such as salt water experiment and phenolphthalein experiment. In salt water experiment, little salt is added to water in a glass container then electrodes attached to direct current terminals are inserted. After this when the intensity is increased then you can see many more bubbles getting evolved at negative electrode or cathode and very few at anode. It's because water is splitted into hydrogen and oxygen ions. Hydrogen being positive ion, gets liberated at cathode and oxygen gets liberated at anode. Considering the water molecule it is obvious that the number of hydrogen atoms will be double than oxygen and hence many more bubbles at cathode are evolved as compared to anode. In case of phenolphthalein experiment, add few drops of phenolphthalein over tissue paper and place the electrodes connected to direct current source over it, then pass the current for some time and then you will see pink colour under negative electrode or cathode (Fig. 3.2).

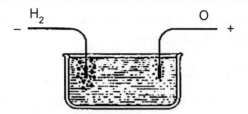

Fig. 3.2: Salt water experiment

PHYSIOLOGICAL EFFECTS

Various physiological effects of direct current are stimulation of sensory nerves, stimulation of motor nerves, accommodation and chemical production.

Stimulation of Sensory Nerves

When direct current is applied to the body tissue, it stimulates sensory nerves and produces burning sensation. This sensory irritation is felt under both the electrodes but if the current flows for sufficient length of time then more irritation is felt under negative electrode.

Stimulation of Motor Nerves

Direct current can produce stimulation of motor nerves during it's on and off. Immediately after direct current is switched on accommodation in motor nerves takes place and hence no further response.

Accommodation

It is physiological adaptation by nerves. Motor nerves get quickly accommodated to direct current and hence it is not possible to stimulate the innervated as well as denervated muscles by direct current. Analogy of accommodation can be done with our feeling of clothes on the body. We feel that we have put-on the clothes after bath but afterwards we get adapted and don't get the same feel throughout the day. Similarly, if one's house is by the main road then he gets used to the night traffic and can have sound sleep as a result of adaptation!

Chemical Production

When direct current is applied to the body tissue it produces chemicals in form of acid and base. Base or alkali is produced at the cathode and acid at the anode. (Remember A for acid and A for anode)

Effect on Body Proteins

It is believed that the direct current causes coagulation of proteins under positive electrode and liquefaction under negative electrode.

THERAPEUTIC INDICATIONS

Therapeutically direct current is used for medical galvanism, anodal galvanism, cathodal galvanism, surgical galvanism and iontophoresis.

Galvanism

Use of direct current without any drug for the treatment of various diseases and disorders is known as galvanism.

Medical Galvanism

Here both the electrodes are of same size. It causes vasomotor stimulation of the skin and increased circulation to the body part where direct current is applied. Medical galvanism is used for acute and chronic inflammatory conditions such as chilblain, Raynaud's disease, Burger's disease, etc.(Fig. 3.3).

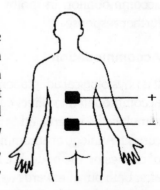

Fig. 3.3: Medical

Anodal Galvanism

Here anode is an active electrode and cathode, which is larger, acts as an indifferent electrode. Anodal galvanism produces acidic reaction, hardens the tissue and reduces nerve irritability. (We will coin a word 'HARN' to remember these effects where H stands for harden, A for acidic reaction and RN for reduce nerve irritability.) Anodal galvanism is used for pain relief (Fig. 3.4).

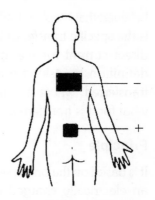

Fig. 3.4: Anodal

Cathodal Galvanism

Here cathode is an active electrode and anode is indifferent electrode. It produces basic reaction or alkaline reaction, softens the tissues and increases nerve irritability. It is used to soften the scar tissue (Fig. 3.5).

Surgical Galvanism or Electrolysis

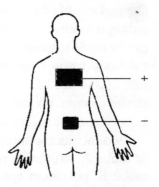

Fig. 3.5: Cathodal

Surgical galvanism or electrolysis is destruction of superfluous hair (hypertrichosis) by the use of galvanic current. Here cathode, which acts as an active electrode is in form of a needle and anode, is indifferent electrode. Half mA of direct current is applied for one minute. Bubble will come out and then hair can be lifted easily with forceps. Aseptic precautions should be taken during this procedure. Skill is required for surgical galvanism. There are 10 to 20% chances of recurrence following this technique.

IONTOPHORESIS

It is also known as ion transfer, ionization or cataphoric medication (Memorize these names with synonym ICI). It is believed that Stephen Leduc discovered it in 1903. Iontophoresis is the specific transfer of ions into the body tissue by the use of direct current for therapeutic purpose. [You can recall this definition by asking questions to yourself such as what is transferred, where it is transferred, how it is transferred, and what for it is transferred.]

Principle

It is based on the principle that an electrically charged electrode will repel a similarly charged ion. In other words, if a drug is in ionic form then it can be made to travel through the body tissue through the skin by the use of direct current via repulsive force between similar charges. We can understand this theory or principle with Leduc experiment (Fig. 3.6).

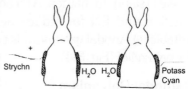

Fig. 3.6: Leduc experiment

Two rabbits are arranged in series. Over positive electrode of rabbit A, strychnine is applied. Over negative electrode of rabbit B, potassium cyanide is applied. Other electrodes are moistened in order to allow the passage of current. Pass direct current through this series arrangement. Rabbit B will die and rabbit A will have convulsions. Place new rabbits and reverse the polarity, there will be no effect. This suggests that there is transfer of ions when placed over similarly charged electrode.

Effectiveness

Effectiveness of iontophoresis depends on number of ions transferred and depth of penetration. Number of ions transferred is determined by current density, duration of current flow and concentration of ions. Iontophoresis is facilitated by increased vasodilatation to the area under electrodes and inhibited by insoluble nature of ions.

Method of Application

Assessment

When you have decided to go for iontophoresis then enquire about allergy to any drug, inspect the area of body where iontophoresis is to be done and check the sensation.

Selection of ion: Select the chemical solution containing the desired ions with adequate concentration. For example if you wanted analgesic effect then select salicylic acid as a solution since it contains salisylate ions which has analgesic properties.

Explain the procedure: Explain the procedure to your patient so that he is aware about what you are going to do and co-operate with you.

Position: Position your patient in such a way that he is comfortable during the treatment. I prefer mostly supine lying.

Clean the area to be treated: Clean the area of body to be treated with spirit or normal saline and cotton swab. It reduces the skin resistance and removes the dust particles from the area and thus facilitates iontophoresis.

Preparation of electrodes and placement: Moisten or soak the piece of bath towel/lint cloth in the drug solution and place it overactive electrode and now place the active electrode over the body part to be treated or massage the solution into the skin and place the active electrode over it. Place the larger indifferent electrode at least 18″ away from the active electrode. Secure the electrodes in position with velcro straps.

Application of treatment: Connect the electrodes to desired terminals. Increase the intensity until prickling, tingling or burning sensation is produced or 0.1to 0.5 mA/cm^2 of electrode. Continue the treatment for 15 minutes and check the undersurface of electrodes after every 5 minutes so as to prevent electrochemical burn.

Termination of the treatment: After 15 minutes reduce intensity gradually and remove the electrodes.

USES OF IONTOPHORESIS

Iontophoresis is commonly used for arthritic and myalgic pain, softening of the scar tissues and adhesions, gouty and calcium deposits, bursitis and tendonitis, hyperhydrosis, wounds and ulcer healing and allergic rhinitis. For the relief of pain and muscle spasm in cases of myalgia, arthritis and sprain, sodium salicylic acid can be used. In order to soften the scar tissue and adhesions sodium chloride solution can be used. Gouty deposits or calcium deposits can be treated with acetic acid iontophoresis. Inflammatory conditions such as bursitis, tendonitis, etc. can be treated with hydrocortisone iontophoresis. Hyperhydrosis, which is characterized by excessive sweating, can be treated with hyloronidase iontophoresis. Iontophoresis for the acceleration of wounds and ulcer healing can be done with zinc sulphate. For acceleration of wounds and ulcers healing, zinc sulphate solution with adequate concentration (5%) is used. Zinc sulphate can also be used to reduce infection such as athlete's foot/tinea pedia and in the treatment of allergic rhinitis. Histamine iontophoresis is used to increase blood supply.

(You can memories these uses with this sentence: SRG All inflammation and infection of wounds ulcers leads to hyperhydrosis. Here you only need to remember that SRG stands for soften scar, relief of pain and gout and 'ALL' for allergic).

Polarity of active electrode	Solution	Ion utilized
Negative	Sodium salicylate	Salicylate
Negative	Sodium chloride	Chloride
Negative	Potassium iodide	Iodide
Negative	Acetic acid	Acetate
Positive	Zinc sulphate	Zinc
Positive	Copper sulphate	Copper
Positive	Wyeth	Hyloronidase
Positive	Decadron	Dexamethasone

CONTRAINDICATIONS AND DANGERS

Various contraindications for iontophoresis are hypersensitivity, impaired sensation and pregnancy. You can remember the contraindications with pneumonic 'HIP' where H stands for hypersensitivity; I stand for impaired sensation and P for pregnancy. Dangers of iontophoresis are chemical burns, alarming shock, electric shock and headache. Chemical burn or tissue destruction is likely to occur if the current density is high, metal electrode touches the skin directly because of insufficient padding. Shock may occur if patient touches the live part of the circuit from which direct current is produced or if the insulation of main cable is defective. Alarming shock is likely to occur if circuit is broken suddenly. It may occur if electrodes are not moistened enough or when wrinkles are present or air gaps are present between electrodes and body tissue. Blood pressure changes/headache: It may occur in case of histamine iontophoresis.

FARADIC CURRENT

Let us understand what is original faradic and faradic type of currents in the beginning so that you can have comprehensive idea about faradic current.

Original Faradic Current

Original faradic current was extensively used in the past. It is a type of current, which can be produced by a faradic coil. Please refer the figure

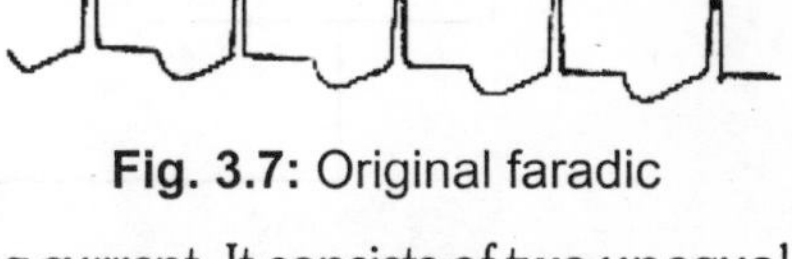

Fig. 3.7: Original faradic

and note that it is an alternating current. It consists of two unequal phases, the first phase is of low intensity and long duration and second phase is of high intensity and short duration. Here second phase is effective and its duration is one millisecond. Frequency of the original faradic current is 50 cycles per second (Fig. 3.7)

Faradic Type Current

This type of current is also called as modern type of current. It is a short durated interrupted direct current with pulse duration of 0.1 to 1msec and a frequency of 50 to100Hz. It is

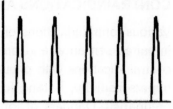

Fig. 3.8: Faradic type

obtained from electronic stimulator. It has got similar physiological effect as that of original faradic current (Fig. 3.8).

PRODUCTION

It is produced on the same principle as that of interrupted direct current. But values of condenser and resistance are low so as to get short duration of impulses and high frequency. An electric pulse generator that produces faradic current has got 4 functional parts in form of power supply, oscillator circuit, modulating circuit and amplifying circuit. Power supply may be from battery or AC. Oscillator circuit provide short duration pulses of 0.1to 1ms with a frequency of 50 to 100Hz. Modulating circuit gives surged out put and amplifying circuit increases the output voltage appropriately (Fig. 3.9).

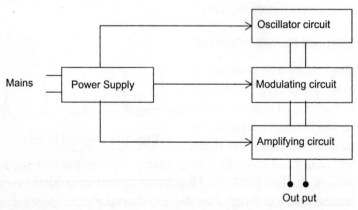

Fig. 3.9: Block diagram of muscle stimulator circuit

INTERRUPTION AND SURGING

Faradic current can be modified by interruption and surging. Hence two forms of modified faradic current can be made available for treatment purpose. Incase of interrupted faradic current the output is interrupted at regular intervals. Generally it is used so as to avoid fatigue of muscles because of higher frequency such as 100Hz (Figs 3.10 and 3.11).

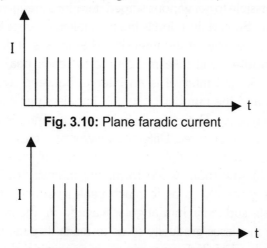

Fig. 3.10: Plane faradic current

Fig. 3.11: Interrupted faradic current

Surged faradic current is a modification of faradic current characterized by gradual increase in the intensity in such a manner that each impulse reaches to higher intensity than that of preceding one and after peak level it either falls suddenly or gradually. Surging is also termed as ramping. Surging is obtained automatically in case of modern stimulators by the use of electronic devices. Advantages of surging are, it avoids fatigue, it does not give surprise to the patient as current slowly increases over the time and not abruptly, contraction of muscle is similar to physiological/ voluntary contraction, avoid or delay the muscle fatigue and avoid elicitation of stretch reflex (Fig. 3.12).

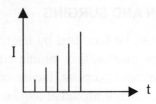

Fig. 3.12: Surged faradic current

It is possible to get various surged durations, frequencies and waveform. Surged duration is the time taken by impulses so as to reach peak level of the intensity. That means, if duration is more, impulses will take more time to reach peak level of intensity. Surged interval is an interval between two surged impulses and the number of surged impulses per unit time is surged frequency. Theoretically frequency of impulses in surged impulses can be adjusted. Different waveforms such as saw tooth, triangular and trapezoidal can be available with surged faradic current. In saw tooth wave form, the intensity of impulses increases gradually so as to reach peak level and after peak level it falls suddenly. In triangular wave form, the intensity of impulses increases gradually so as to reach its peak level and after peak level it falls down gradually. In trapezoidal, the intensity of impulses increased gradually so as to reach peak level, at peak level it remains for some time and then it falls gradually.

PHYSIOLOGICAL EFFECTS

Physiological effects of original faradic and faradic type of current are stimulation of sensory nerves, stimulation of motor nerves, effect of muscle contraction, increased metabolism, effect on denervated muscle and chemical effect.

Stimulation of Sensory Nerves

When faradic type of current is applied to the body then there is feeling of mild prickling sensation as a result of stimulation of sensory nerves. Stimulation of sensory nerves also causes reflex vasodilatation of superficial blood vessel leading to reddening of the skin or erythema.

Stimulation of Motor Nerves

Faradic type of current stimulates motor nerves and if intensity is sufficient then it will cause contraction of muscles supplied by it. As stimulations are repeated 50 times per second or more than that and hence it produces tetanic contraction. If this type of contraction is continued for more than a short period of time then muscle fatigue is produced and hence, the current is surged or interrupted in order to give relaxation. Advantage of surging is strength of contraction increases gradually in such a manner that is similar to voluntary contraction.

Chemical Effect

Very negligible amount of chemicals are formed when faradic current is applied, as the pulse duration is too small.

Effect on Denervated Muscle

Faradic current is never used for stimulation of denervated muscle. Since the intensity of current required for producing a contraction of denervated muscle with a faradic current is usually too great to be tolerable for the treatment purposes. Therefore, the faradic current is not satisfactory for the stimulation of denervated muscles.

Effect of Muscle Contraction

Electrical stimulation of muscles by faradic current increases metabolism and pumping effect of muscles. Metabolism is a collective process, which consists of physical, chemical, anabolic and catabolic changes in the body tissues by which living state of body is maintained. As a result of muscle contraction due to electrical stimulation, metabolism is increased. Increased metabolism increases demand for oxygen and foodstuffs and as a result of it; there is increase in the output of waste products including metabolites. These metabolites cause dilation of capillaries and arterioles and increase the blood supply to the muscle.

As the muscle contract and relax it exert a pumping action on veins, lymphatic vessels lying within and around them. The valves in this vessel direct the fluid towards the heart. If muscle contraction is strong and joint movement is also there then both of these exert a pumping effect on vessels leading to increased venous and lymphatic return.

THERAPEUTIC INDICATIONS

Faradic current is primarily used to produce contraction of normally innervated muscles and current is usually surged so as to get contractions, which resembles to voluntary contractions.

Facilitation of Muscle

Muscle contraction can be facilitated by faradic type of current. The facilitation effect of faradic current can be used when a patient is unable to produce a muscle contraction or finds difficulty in doing so. Muscle contraction may be inhibited as a result trauma, inflammation, pain and surgery, etc. (you can remember with a word TIPS). Here faradic current stimulation is used in assisting voluntary contraction, for example faradic stimulation of quadriceps following menisectomy. Patient should be encouraged to attempt voluntary contraction at the same time so as to get voluntary control.

Muscle Re-education

Muscle action can be re-educated if voluntary muscle action is lost as a result of prolonged disease or incorrect use. For instance re-education of abductor hallucis in hallux valgus. Here the current is applied in such a way that it produces the abduction of great toe.

New Muscle Action

After tendon transplantation or other reconstruction operations, faradic current can be used for training of new muscle action. Muscle is stimulated so as to produce the new action or movement. During stimulation, patient should attempt to perform voluntary contraction. Once the patient is able to perform new movement actively without electric stimulation then electric stimulation is discontinued.

Motor Nerve Neurapraxia

Faradic stimulation to the paralyzed muscles can be applied following neurapraxic lesion of the motor nerve. Electrical stimulation can be given till voluntary control is developed. However, electrical stimulation may not be needed in neurapraxia as recovery takes place without any marked changes in the muscle tissue.

Blood Supply

Faradic current can cause reflex vasodilatation and hence can be used for increase in blood supply in conditions, where heat treatment may not be a safer choice. For this purpose sensory level intensity is applied with bath method of application.

Effect on Edema

Faradic current can be used in the treatment of edema for improving venous and lymphatic drainage. Faradism under pressure method of faradic current application can be used for this purpose.

USES OF FARADIC CURRENT

Faradic current can be used in the treatment of muscle inhibition, edema, incontinence, hallux valgus, Bell's palsy (neurapraxic lesion), metatarsalgia, postural flat feet, after tendoachillis surgery, after knee surgeries, rheumatoid arthritis, tendon transplantation, later stages of peripheral nerve injuries, chillblain, muscle spasm, pain relief by counter-irritation, etc.

METHODS OF APPLICATION

Faradic current can be applied by various methods such as motor point stimulation, labile, stabile, nerve conduction method, bath method, under pressure faradism, etc.

Motor Point Stimulation

It involves stimulation of individual muscle. In this method an indifferent electrode is placed at the origin of muscle and an active disc electrode (handle/pen electrode) is placed at motor point. With this method almost each and every muscle can be stimulated and thus effect of passive exercise can be given to each and every muscle. However, it is somewhat difficult to stimulate deeply situated muscles with this method. Advantages of this method are, contraction of individual muscle can be obtained, each and every muscle can be stimulated and isolated muscle contraction can be obtained in the treatment of various conditions for example stimulation of abductor hallucis in hallux valgus. However, there are some disadvantages of this method such as it is tedious, time consuming, trial error method and it's difficult to stimulate the deeply situated muscle (You can remember them with 3T deep).

Labile Method

This method can be used for stimulation of large muscles with multiple nerve supply for example trunk muscles. Here an indifferent electrode is placed at origin of muscle or muscles and an active electrode in form of either disc or small plate electrode is moved over area to be treated. During this method current is not usually surged. As the active electrode approach and leave motor point of a muscle, that muscle contracts and relaxes respectively.

Nerve Conduction Method

In this method an indifferent electrode is placed at convenient area and an active electrode to a point at which the nerve trunk is superficial. It will stimulate motor nerve trunk and will cause contractions of all the muscles that it supplies beyond the point of stimulation. This method is used when it is not possible to use other methods conveniently for example in case of wound, splint and edema.

Bath Method

Application of faradic current to the body parts in a tub, tray or tank containing water is termed as bath method of application. Depending upon placement of electrodes bath can be of bipolar or unipolar type. In bipolar, both electrodes are kept in bath and in case of unipolar, only one electrode is kept in the bath while the other one is kept at any convenient part of the body, which is not immersed in the water. Bath method is commonly used for the application of faradic current to the foot and which is often termed as faradic footbath. Advantages of bath method are that skin resistance is lowered considerably by water and in addition to this water makes perfect contact with the tissues. Disadvantages of this method of application are that the current can not be localized, superficial muscles contract to a greater extent than deeper ones and due to the presence of water, chances of electric shock is greater as water can make earthing easily available.

Faradism Under Pressure

This method is used in the treatment of edema to increase the venous and lymphatic drainage from the edematous area. Here the faradic current is applied along with an elastic bandage such as elastocerepe bandage and the body part, which is to be treated, is kept elevated during the treatment. This form of treatment is applied for 15 to 20 minutes only.

Faradism to Pelvic Floor Muscles

Here the active electrode is placed in the perineal region or rectum or vagina and an indifferent electrode over lumbosacral region. This method of application can be used in prolapse of pelvic organs, stress incontinence, etc.

INTERRUPTED DIRECT CURRENT

Interrupted direct current is also known as modified direct current or interrupted galvanic current. Interrupted direct current is commonly used for stimulation of denervated muscles and for electrodiagnostic purpose. It is a modified type of direct current characterized by commencement and cessation of the current flow at regular intervals. In other words, it is a current whose flow stops and starts at regular intervals. Impulse duration ranges between 0.01msec to 3000 msec and the frequency vary as per the pulse duration and the interval selected between them, for instance if the impulse duration is 100 millisecond then the frequency is 30 cycles per second. The pulses used in interrupted direct current can be called as long durated and short durated pulses. Long durated pulses are those whose duration is more than 10 millisecond and short durated are those whose duration is less than 10 millisecond. Various waveforms of interrupted direct current such as saw tooth, triangular, depolarized, trapezoidal and rectangular can be used in clinical applications. (Memorize with ST, DTR It's not standard deep tendon reflex! But it is saw tooth, triangular, depolarized, trapezoidal and rectangular) (Fig. 3.13).

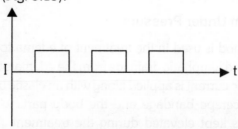

Fig. 3.13: Interrupted direct current

Production

Interrupted direct current for the treatment can be availed from battery or electricity operated stimulator. Electronic muscle stimulator works on multivibrator or flip flap circuit. Refer the figure 3.9 for more details.

Physiological and Therapeutic Effects

Physiological effects of interrupted direct current are stimulation of sensory nerves, stimulation of motor nerves, effect of muscle contraction, increased metabolism, effect on denervated muscle and chemical effect.

Sensory Nerve Stimulation

When interrupted direct current is applied to the body then there is feeling of stabbing or burning sensation as a result of stimulation of sensory nerves. Stimulation of sensory nerves also causes reflex vasodilatation of superficial blood vessel leading to reddening of the skin or erythema.

Motor Nerve Stimulation

Interrupted direct current stimulates motor nerves and if intensity is sufficient then it will cause contraction of muscles supplied by it. It produces very brisk contraction followed by immediate relaxation of innervated muscles but sluggish contraction of denervated muscles if the impulse duration is adequate. Sluggish contraction means worm like slow contraction and relaxation. Since interrupted direct current can produce the contractions of denervated muscles, it is commonly used in the treatment of peripheral nerve injuries to stimulate the muscles so as to prevent or minimize the possibility of atrophy, degeneration and fibrosis of muscles following denervation. (Remember it with FAD: fibrosis, atrophy and degeneration). However, it should be remembered that therapeutic electrical stimulation does not accelerate the rate of regeneration following peripheral nerve injuries or neuropathies (Fig. 3.14).

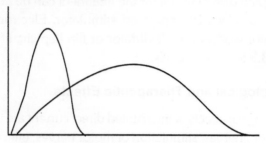

Fig. 3.14: Brisk and sluggish contraction

Effect on Denervated Muscle

Following denervation muscles undergo various changes. These changes include paralysis, flaccidity; atrophy, decreased muscle weight, decreased muscle protein, decreased sarcoplasm, decrease in number of muscle fibers, replacement by fibrous and adipose tissues, and degeneration. Stimulation of denervated muscle improves its nutrition by increasing the blood supply. Blood supply is increased due to muscle contractions as a result of pumping effect. As a result of electrical stimulation nutrition of muscles is improved and which in turn retards atrophy, degeneration and fibrosis. For this purpose electrical stimulation can be applied to produce 90 contractions of each muscle every day. But this is controversial; various trends followed are 10 to 30 contractions, 30 to 300 contractions per day or three times per week. I personally feel that these variations are as per the convenience of the therapist and patients!

Chemical Effect

Very negligible amount of chemicals are formed when interrupted direct current is applied since there is pause or rest in between any two impulses.

As the muscle contract and relax it exert a pumping action on veins, lymphatic vessels lying within and around them. The valves in these vessels direct the fluid towards the heart. If muscle contraction is strong and moreover there is joint movement then both of these exert a pumping effect on vessels leading to increase venous and lymphatic return.

Pole Used for Stimulation

Usually cathode is used as an active electrode but sometimes a greater response can be obtained to anode and hence, it should be decided on the basis of clinical situation as per the response to these poles in denervated muscles.

Uses and Methods of Applications

Interrupted direct current is used in the treatment of denervated muscles and for elecetrodiagnostic tests such as strength duration curves, faradic interrupted direct current test, pulse ratio, etc. Interrupted direct current can also be used for healing purpose. For this purpose sub sensory thresholds have been used and this is termed as low intensity direct current therapy (LIDC). Methods of application commonly used in the treatment with interrupted direct current are motor point, stabile and labile.

TRANSCUTANEOUS ELECTRICAL NERVE STIMULATION

It is a form of peripheral electrical nerve stimulation through the skin, which is used to obtain electroanalgesia. In past, TENS equipments were also used as nerve tracers for the search of percutaneous nerves, for maintenance of muscle activity after the stroke and for muscle development. Today, TENS is one of the most commonly used electrotherapeutic modality for the pain relief.

Historical Aspects

In the first century AD Scriborius Largus described the use of electrical shocks for the relief of chronic pain. The Roman and

Greek physicians have reported the use of certain species of fish for pain relief such as Torpedo mamorata, Malapterus and Gymnotus electricus who had an organ that produces electric charges. Typically the fish was kept in contact with the area of the body experiencing pain to produce series of electrical shocks. These crude methods continued until mid 18th century. During 1745 Leyden jar was introduced and the same was used as power source for electroanalgesia. During the 19th century the development of battery and induction coil added further sophistication. Introduction of electroanalgesia into the medical profession was met with considerable skepticism and inevitable opposition to this concept.   Due to this and variable clinical results there was decline in the interest towards the end of 19th century in the use of electrical stimulation as a means of pain relief. In addition to this, in 20th century the increased number of analgesics turned the interest away from the use of peripheral stimulation as a pain-relieving mode. But in 1965 Ronald Melzac and Patric Wall published their gate control theory and hence, the interest again reawakened in the use of electrical stimulation as a pain-relieving mode. During same period (1960s) dorsal column stimulators were introduced. Dorsal column stimulators involved the surgical implantation of electrodes in dorsal column of spinal cord, which were activated by an external battery operated device. Dr. Norman Shealy initially used battery-operated device as a screening device to establish the patient's candidacy for dorsal column stimulator implantation surgery. If the patients responded favorably to such external transcutaneous stimulation then this was taken as an indication that they would respond positively to dorsal column stimulator. But he (Norman Shealy) noted that some of his patients responded better to transcutaneous stimulation than to dorsal column stimulation and so TENS was discovered almost accidentally. This discovery initiated a new era for electroanalgesia. Meyer and Fields (1972) were the first to report clinical use of TENS for the relief chronic pain. In the following years, researchers and manufacturers combinely developed several types of TENS devices with a range of adjustable parameters.

Characteristics

Frequency   In conventional TENS it is 10 to100 Hz and in modern TENS it may vary from 2 to 600Hz. Frequency is adjustable in both the types of TENS equipments (Fig. 3.15).

Pulse width   Pulse with varies from 50 to 300 microseconds. Pulse width is also adjustable.

Pulse shape   Pulse shape is usually modified rectangular.

Output of intensity   It varies from 0 to 60 milliamperes.

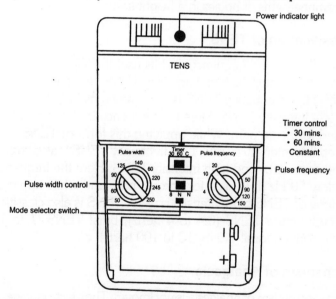

Fig. 3.15: Portable TENS device

Modulation of TENS

It is believed that the body tissues may get accommodated to TENS current and hence to prevent this, TENS current is modulated. Gradual and continuous change in one or more than one parameters of TENS current in order to prevent accommodation is known as TENS modulation. It can be brought about by changes in frequency or pulse width or amplitude or all together. Usually 10% modulation is used. Frequency modulation is characterized by gradual and continuous changes in frequency. For example, if modulated frequency is selected, as 100Hz then frequency will gradually vary from 90 to100 in a manner like 90, 91, 92... 100 and once again same trend will be continued. In pulse width modulation there will be gradual and continuous changes in pulse width. In amplitude modulation there is continuous and automatic variation in amplitude. In burst modulation the output is in form of groups of stimuli ranging from one to ten. And in train modulation the output is similar to the arrangements of bogies in a freight train.

Classification of TENS

Depending on the frequency and its use, the TENS is divided into two types such as high frequency TENS and low frequency TENS. High frequency TENS is also known as high frequency and low intensity TENS. Here the frequency is above 50 Hz. It is used for acute pain. While applying this form of TENS only perceptible intensity is used. Low frequency TENS is also known as low frequency and high intensity TENS. Here the frequency is below 50 Hz. It is used for chronic pain and while applying this type of TENS high intensity is used. TENS is also classified as acupuncture TENS (0.4 to 4 hertz), burst TENS (1 to 10 hertz), conventional TENS (10 to 100 hertz), etc.

Mechanism of Analgesia

Exact mechanism of analgesia is not known. The electroanalgesia by TENS may occur as per the Endorphin theory or Gate control theory.

Endorphin Theory

TENS causes stimulation and increase in circulation of endorphins. Endorphins are morphine like endogenous transmitter substances. They occur naturally in brain and pituitary glands. Endorphins from the brain circulate and block the pain sensation as a result of TENS application.

Gate Control Theory

Dr. Ronald Melzac and Patrick Wall described the gate control theory in 1965 to explain the mechanism of analgesia. Theme of this theory is, pain may be blocked at various gates through which pain impulse travels to the brain. These gates are located at neuronal synapses in the spinal cord.

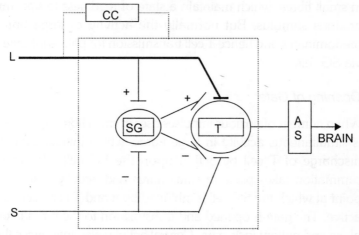

Fig. 3.16: Gate control theory
In figure, L: large diameter nerve fiber which carries proprioceptive impulses mainly, S: small diameter nerve fiber which mainly carries pain impulses, SG: substantia gelatinosa, T: transmission cell, AS: activating system and CC: central control.

Information leading to pain generation passes through gate and depends upon the balance activity in large and small afferent nerve fibres and in the fibres descending down from higher centers. The transmission of pain sensation depends upon the activation of the transmission cell (T) by large or small nerve fibres. The amount of transmission from these fibres to the T cell is governed intern by the action of a further cell in substantia gelatinosa of spinal cord (SG). It produces its effect by presynaptic and postsynaptic inhibition. SG cell is activated from the collateral branches from large fibres, chiefly those ascending in the dorsal columns of spinal cord dealing with proprioception and touch. It is inhibited by small fiber activity namely those known to be concerned with pain generation.

Normal Circumstances

In normal circumstances there is low but constant rate of activity in small fibres, which maintain a state of readiness to transmit noxious stimulus. But normally the activity of large fibres predominates and hence T cell transmission for pain is inhibited via SG cell.

Opening of Gate

When number of noxious impulses rises in small fibres then there is simultaneous activity in large fibres, which initially inhibits discharge of T cell by action upon the SG cell. However, summation takes place in small fibres and activity reaches a point at which the SG cell is inhibited by it and T cell becomes active. The gate is opened and transmission to the brain takes place and patient feels pain. Central activity also influences the situation, thus it may facilitate or inhibit pain information. For example in heightened anxiety, the level of pain is increased, as it seems that activity generated in the limbic system of brain and transmitted via reticular formation of brain stem results in opening of gate. On the other hand, pain may not be experienced while an individual is engaged in sporting contest. Perhaps it may be due to inhibitory effects of higher centers, which closes the gate.

TENS and Closing of Gate

Stimulation of large nerve fibres by TENS activate SG cell and inhibit the discharge of T cell probably by its effect via presynaptic or postsynaptic inhibition. This closes the gate and causes analgesia. The duration for which this gate remains closed varies and is directly proportional to the number of noxious impulses in small fibres.

NaK Pump and Pain Relief by TENS

Repetitive antidromic stimulation of postsynaptic axon can alter extra cellular potassium ion concentration and reduces the excitatory postsynaptic potential.

INDICATIONS

TENS is used commonly for electroanalgesia in enormous conditions.

Joint pain: Rheumatoid arthritis, osteoarthritis, intraarticular hemorrhage, etc.

Acute pain: It can also be used in the treatment of the acute pain such as obstetric or labor pain, acute trauma, acute orofacial pain, postoperative pain, and primary dysmenorrhea.

Muscle pain: It is also used in the treatment of pain due to various muscle disorders such as muscle spasm, spastic torticollis, myositis, myalgia, and muscle strain.

Spinal pain: spinal cord injury, dorsal root compression syringomyelitis, arachanoiditis, post cordotomy, spinal nerve compression, can be very well treated.

Neoplastic pain: It can be used in the treatment of neoplasic conditions. In severe neoplasic pain, TENS can be used for 24 hours a day with a portable device. It can be applied with self-adhesive electrodes so that patient can perform his ADL while receiving TENS.

Nerve disorders: peripheral nerve injuries, traumatic neuromas, trigeminal neuralgia, causalgia, brachial neuralgia, intercostals neuritis, mononeuritis, polyneuritis and neuropathies.

Miscellaneous conditions: itch, angina pectoris, functional abdominal pain and pancreatitis.

Non-analgesics indications: TENS can also be used in dysmenorrhea, Raynaud's disease, Burger's disease, wound healing and following reconstructive surgeries.

Psychogenic and phantom pain: These pains also can be treated with TENS.

CONTRAINDICATIONS AND PRECAUTIONS

The beauty of the TENS modality is there are very few contraindications such as anesthesia or sensory loss and demand type of cardiac pacemaker. However, precautions should be taken while applying the TENS in case of pregnancy, area of carotid sinus, area of mouth, on the eyelids, epileptic patients, in patients with arrhythmias or myocardial disease, undiagnosed pain (since it can mask the important diagnostic symptom). Keep the TENS device out of reach of children. There are no side effects except skin irritation, which may occur sometime. To prevent it, it is necessary to wash the area of application and electrode following the treatment.

Electrode Placement in TENS

Various electrodes such as carbon impregnated, silicon rubber or pad electrodes can be used for TENS applications. Carbon electrodes or silicon rubber electrodes of various sizes can be used as per the requirement. Three sizes such as 45X45, 45X95, and 45X190 mm are commonly used. But the choice of the size varies on the extent of the area to be treated. Carbon or silicon rubber electrodes can be kept in good contact with the skin with the help of electroconductive gel. Electrodes are usually placed over spinal cord segment, acupuncture point, over painful dermatome, over and around painful area, over nerve trunk, over tender spot and over trigger points. (You can memorize these sites by the word SAD ANTT! Where S for spinal segment, A for area of pain, D for dermatome, A for acupuncture, N for nerve trunk, T for tender spot and T for trigger point).

Dosiometry

In acute pain, high frequency and low or perceptible intensity TENS can be applied for 20 minutes and in chronic pain low frequency TENS can be applied with high or tolerable intensity for 30 minutes. However, if the intensity of pain is very severe then TENS can even be applied for 8 to 24 hours!

Benefits of TENS

Due to reduced pain exercise programme can be progressed, activities of daily living may be improved, faster reduction in pain facilitates early return to work, there is no side effects with TENS, TENS reduces cost of medications, early ambulation in postoperative cases can be achieved, TENS is noninvasive, non-toxic and nonpharmacological.

INTERFERENTIAL CURRENT

It is the production of low frequency current in the body tissue by the simultaneous application of two different medium frequency currents. As it is obtained as a result of interference of two different medium frequency currents, it is known as interferential current. Alternatively interferential current can be defined as the resultant current produced in the body tissue when two medium frequency alternating currents are applied simultaneously. This current is produced at the intersection of two medium frequency alternating currents. Historically in 1950 H. Nemac for the first time suggested interferential current for therapeutic application. It is also called as Russian currents as Dr. KM Kots first described its use in 1970 in the Russian literature.

CHARACTERISTICS

Before reading the characteristics please refer the Figure 3.17 for the sake of comprehension.

Currents

Two medium frequency currents are used to produce the interferential current. They are known as carrier waves as they do not produce muscle nerve stimulation and are just used to get the greater depth of penetration and to produce the interferential current. Out of two medium frequency currents the frequency of one current is fixed and it is 4000 hertz. The frequency of the other current lies in between 4000 to 4100 hertz, which is adjustable. When these currents crosses each other they will produce a third current at the point where they crosses each other and this third current is known as interferential current (Fig. 3.17).

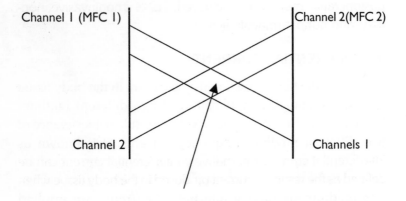

Fig. 3.17: Interferential current

Beat Frequency

The frequency of the resultant current (third current produced due to crossing) is known as beat frequency. Beat frequency is equal to the difference between two medium frequency currents. It lies between 0 to 100 hertz. Beat frequency may be kept constant or varied rhythmically so as to prevent accommodation. Constant beat frequency is also called as selective beat frequency. Different selective beat frequencies can be selected in between 0 to 100 hertz.

Variable Beat Frequency

It is also called as automatic beat frequency. Various variable beat frequencies can be used. Beat frequency of 0 to 5 hertz stimulate sympathetic nerves, 5 to 10 hertz stimulate parasympathetic nerves, 10 to 50 hertz stimulate motor nerves, 50 to 90 hertz produces sedative and spasmolytic effect and 90 to 100 hertz produces analgesic or pain relief effect. (Memory cue, SPM, SP social and preventive medicine's special portion!! where S=sympathetic, P= parasympathetic, M=motor nerves, S= spasmolytic, and P= pain relief).

Area of Interference

It is the area where interferential current is set-up. The pattern of the interferential area may be static or dynamic. I would like you to refer the Figure 3.18 before reading further.

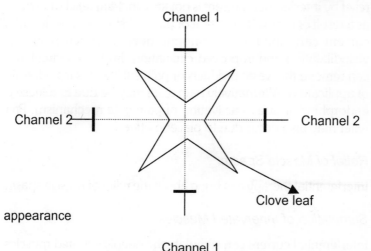

Fig. 3.18: Area of interference

Static Interference

Here the area in which interferential current is set-up remains stationary. This area of static interference gives an appearance of clove leaf as a result of the vector addition of two currents and it lies to 45° angles to the perpendicular lines from each electrode.

Dynamic Area of Interference

It is possible to move the area in which interference current is developed in a to and fro manner through 45°. It is obtained by varying the current intensity in suitable manner. Current is varied from 50 to 100%. This dynamic area of interference is also called as vector sweep, vector scan, rotating vector, etc.

THERAPEUTIC EFFECTS

Pain Relief

Interferential current is commonly used for electro-analgesia in various musculoskeletal conditions. Exact mechanism of pain relief by interferential current is not known. Pain relief may occur as a result of removal of irritant or pain substances. Interferential current can stimulate autonomic nerves, which results in vasodilatation and improved circulation. Improved circulation can remove the waste products or pain substances from the site of application. Alternatively pain relief may be due to release of endorphins or due to activation of pain gate mechanism. Pain relief may also occur due to placebo effect.

Relief of Muscle Spasm

Interferential therapy can bring about the relief of muscle spasm.

Stimulation of Innervated Muscles

Interferential current can stimulate the deeply situated muscles, as it is like a low frequency current.

Effect on Edema

Interferential current can improve the drainage of blood and lymph. This effect can be used in the treatment of edema.

Electrodes

In electrotherapy, electrodes are the conductors, which are used to allow the easy passage of therapeutic currents to the body. Various types of electrodes can be used for the application of interferential current; such as vacuum electrode, pad electrode, carbon impregnated/silicon rubber electrode, four field electrodes, two field double electrodes, quadripolar /four point probe electrode, labile electrode, etc.

Vacuum Electrode

Vacuum electrode is like a rubber bell. Here the electrode is kept at the base of bell and wire or lead is connected at narrow end. Generally a soaked sponge or spontex is kept just below the electrode so as to achieve even contact to skin and hence better conduction. These electrodes are held to the patient with negative pressure created by a vacuum pump. The magnitude of the vacuum should be adjusted so that the least amount of suction is necessary to keep the electrodes on the skin otherwise superficial bruising may occur. Vacuum electrodes are available in various sizes. Vacuum can be adjusted so as to get constant or pulsed mode. When pulsed mode is used then additional effect of massage can be obtained. Vacuum electrodes are excellent for treating flat smooth areas where they can be applied easily and quickly. On bony areas such as shoulder and ankle, it is difficult to place the vacuum cup in correct position without deformation. The deformation squeezes the cup and area enclosed by rim is diminished. As a result of the deformation the two electrodes in a particular channel would not be of the same size and the circuit is unbalanced. On hairy skin it is difficult to get an airtight seal. In elderly patients the skin is likely to be thin and papery, it presents difficulty with contact and bruise easily. Vacuum electrodes are considered unsafe for patients who are taking steroids because of likelihood of bruising.

Labile Electrodes

It is a special type of plate electrode, which is insulated on one side and is covered with sponge to provide contact. Two electrodes are used for the treatment purpose. The operator holds them in position while treating. During the treatment, these electrodes are moved over the patient's skin. Usually one side of the electrode is insulated or operator put-on the gloves so that current does not passes through the operator's hand while applying the current through these electrodes to the patient. Then operator secures them to his palms with velcro. It is helpful if foot control is available otherwise both the electrodes are first held by one hand while the other hand adjusts current. Pads are moved in see saw movement. It is useful in the treatment of muscular conditions and awkward areas.

Dosiometry

Interferential therapy can be applied for 10 to 20 minutes for 10 to 25 days on once a day basis.

Usually the intensity, which produce a strong but comfortable prickling sensations without any discomfort is used. Alternatively three times toleration dose (TTT Dose) can be used. Three T dose is used in treating localized condition that is tender and is to be an anesthetized. Place the electrodes, increase the intensity so as to give intense prickling, once the intense prickling sensation is reduced, increase the intensity once again so as to get intense prickling and repeat the same once again so as to treat the area three times with strong prickling.

Indications

Interferential therapy is commonly used for the pain relief, relief of muscle spasm, improve the venous and lymphatic drainage, and re-education of deeply situated muscles, which are not easily accessible with low frequency currents. Various conditions in which interferential current may be used are; osteoarthritis, ankylosing spondylitis, spondylosis, low back pain, frozen shoulder, chondromalacia, stress incontinence, nocturnal incontinence, brachial neuralgia, sciatica, phantom pain, Burger's disease, Raynaud's disease, myalgia/myositis, edema, following immobilization, bronchial asthma, bursitis, tendonitis, etc.

Contraindications and Precautions

Interferential current is contraindicated in patients with cardiac pacemaker, advanced cardiac disease, hypertension, hypotension, thrombosis, recent haemorrhage, pregnancy, neoplasm, tuberculosis, fever and infection. Interferential apparatus must be kept at least six meters distance away from a short wave diathermy machine, preferably in another room, otherwise circuit damage can occur or the patient may experience a sudden surge of current when the short wave diathermy machine is turned off. To prevent the interference from short wave diathermy a filter circuit can be used in interferential therapy machine.

Methods of Application

Interferential current can be applied by means of bipolar, quadripolar, stereo dynamic and labile method. In bipolar method only two electrodes are used. It is said that in case of bipolar method, medium frequency currents are added to give an output similar to interferential current. This mode of treatment is sometimes known as electrokinesy. In qaudripolar method four electrodes are used. In stereo dynamic systems three pairs of electrodes are used and the machine provides three out puts. It reduces accommodation and provides three-dimensional interferential field. In labile method two labile electrodes are used for the treatment purpose and operator moves them during the treatment.

Advantages of Interferential Current

Interferential current do not produce any sensorimotor irritation, metal is not contraindicated for interferential therapy and hence number of postoperative conditions can be treated with interferential therapy. Interferential current is useful in treating tissues at a greater depth, owing to the frequency the skin resistance is very less, and current can be localized more effectively in specific areas.

SINUSOIDAL CURRENT

It is an evenly alternating, biphasic low frequency current whose waveform resembles to sine curve. Its frequency is 50 to 100 Hz and pulse duration is 10 ms. Sinusoidal current is classified on the basis of frequency as slow sinusoidal and rapid sinusoidal current. Frequency of slow sinusoidal current is 50 Hz and rapid sinusoidal current's frequency is 100 Hz. Practically sinusoidal current resembles to faradic current both in effects as well as methods of application. Nowadays, it is rarely used for the treatment purpose (Fig. 3.19).

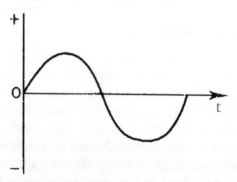

Fig. 3.19: Sinusoidal current

HIGH VOLTAGE PULSED GALVANIC CURRENT

HVPG was popularized in 1970s. Here the current is not truly galvanic. It is monophasic twin peaked high intensity current with pulse duration less than 20 microseconds. (You can memorize monophasic twin peaked high intensity pulsed direct current with MTP, HIPDC) Intensity of 500 volts or 2500 milliampere is used

with this current. Higher intensity of the
current overcomes the natural resistance
of the skin and hence deeper
penetration. Advantages of HVPG are
it reduces the skin resistance, it can
penetrate to deeper tissues, HVPG have
probe electrodes for the treatment and
hence it can be used for the treatment of

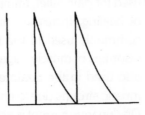

Fig. 3.20: HVPG

trigger points, short pulse width improves the patient comfort and
it produces polarizing effect, although it is smaller but it may be
beneficial in wound healing (Fig. 3.20).

MICROAMPERAGE ELECTRICAL NERVE STIMULATION

Microamperage electrical nerve stimulation (MENS) is a form
of electrotherapy current that provides sub-threshold or
subliminal stimulation. The amplitude of this current is less than
one milliampere, which is insufficient to depolarize sensory and
motor nerves and hence patient does not experience either
tingling sensation or muscle contractions. MENS works on Arndt
Schulz law. According to this law weak stimuli increases
physiologic activity and very strong stimuli inhibit or abolish the
activity. It is believed that MENS increases cell permeability,
increases intracellular concentration of calcium ions, increases
fibroblast activity and increase protein synthesis. Pain relief by
MENS may occur due to reduction in the liberation of pain
producing substances at cellular level. For pain relief purpose
MENS can be applied for ten minutes initially with positive
polarity and later on by negative polarity.

DIADYNAMIC CURRENT

Diadynamic currents are also called as Bernard currents. It is
unidirectional sinusoidal current with a frequency of 50 to 100
Hz and pulse duration 10 milliseconds. Diadynamic current is

used for pain relief, minimizes inflammation, swelling, facilitation of healing, increased circulation and motor re-education. It is commonly used in the treatment of painful and inflammatory disorders of muscles, ligaments, joints and peripheral nerves. It is also used in the treatment of contusion, haematoma, myalgia, muscle atrophy due to immobilization, inactivity and epicondylitis. Diadynamic current is applied for ten minutes once or twice daily with perceptible intensity. Various modulations of diadynamic currents are fix monophase, fix diaphase, short periods and long periods, syncopated rhythm and modulated monophase.

SUMMARY

Muscle nerve stimulating currents are used primarily for muscle re-education, pain relief and to delay atrophy and wasting of muscle. Various currents included in this category are direct current, faradic current, interrupted direct current, TENS, interferential current, sinusoidal current, diadynamic current, high voltage pulsed galvanic current and MENS. Direct current is unidirectional continuous current. Faradic current is primarily used to produce contraction of normally innervated muscles and current is usually surged so as to get contractions that resembles to voluntary contractions.

Interrupted direct current is commonly used for stimulation of denervated muscles and for electrodiagnostic purpose. TENS is used mainly for pain relief and it is believed that the body tissues may get accommodated to TENS current and hence to prevent this, TENS current is modulated. Interferential current is the production of low frequency current in the body tissue by the simultaneous application of two different medium frequency currents. Practically sinusoidal current resembles to faradic current both in effects as well as methods of application. HVPG is monophasic twin peaked high intensity current with pulse duration less than 20 microseconds. Diadynamic currents are also called as Bernard currents.

chapter four

Diagnostic Electrotherapy

In addition to the therapy, electrical currents can be used for diagnostic purposes. Electrodiagnosis means the detection of the electrical reaction of muscles and nerves for diagnosis, prognosis and therapy by the use of electrotherapeutic currents or electromyography. We can use currents like interrupted direct current and perform various electrodiagnostic tests such as: rheobase, chronaxie, strength duration curve, pulse ratio, galvanic tetanic ratio, nerve conduction test, nerve distribution test, faradic galvanic test, myotonic reaction, reaction of degeneration, etc. When there is disease or injury of motor nerves or muscles, alterations are likely to occur in their response to electrical stimulation. The altered reactions to electrical stimulation may be of considerable assistance in diagnosis of the lesion.

RHEOBASE AND CHRONAXIE

Rheobase

Rheobase is the smallest amount of current required to produce a muscle contraction with a stimulus of infinite duration. Usually impulse of 100ms duration is used to find out the rheobase for practical purpose. Denervation of muscles reduces rheobase and hence it may be less than that of innervated muscles. However, it may increase if reinnervation commences.

Chronaxie

Chronaxie is the shortest duration of electrical impulse that will produce a response with a current of double the rheobase. The chronaxie of the denervated muscles is higher than the innervated muscles. The innervated muscle's chronaxie is 1msec if constant voltage stimulator is used. Chronaxie is not a satisfactory method in case of partial denervation. In such case, chronaxie will be of predominant fibers that are innervated or denervated. Say in case of 75% denervation chronaxie will be same as that of completely denervated muscle.

STRENGTH DURATION CURVES

Definition

It is an electrodiognostic procedure characterized by plotting a graph of amount of intensity required against various durations of impulses so as to determine the status of innervations of muscles. It is also called as intensity time curve.

Apparatus and Other Requirements

A diagnostic muscle stimulator is used for plotting strength duration curve. For this purpose apparatus should provide different durations of interrupted direct current for example, 0.01, 0.03, 0.1, 0.3, 1, 3, 10, 30, 50, 100 and 300 milliseconds with rectangular waveform. Stimulator with either constant voltage or constant current can be used for this purpose. In addition to this electrodes, leads, velcro straps, cotton swabs, water or normal saline, graph paper, pencil and eraser are required for strength duration curve plotting.

Procedure

Procedure for plotting of the strength duration curve can be described in stepwise manner.

Preparation of Patient

Explain the procedure in brief to the patient. Position the patient in a comfortable position, which allow you an easy access to the body part where you would like to perform the strength duration curve assessment. Request your patient to expose the area to be examined and ensure adequate draping. Make sure that there is adequate light to see the visible contractions of muscle without straining your eyes.

Application of Electrodes

Secure the indifferent electrode at a convenient area, usually over mid line of the body or origin of muscle and active electrode over motor point.

Application of Current and Recording

Switch on the stimulator then select the longest impulse say 300 msec and increase the intensity so as to get minimal contraction. This minimal contraction may be assessed visually or by palpation of the tendon. Note the intensity of current required to produce minimal contraction and then decrease the intensity to zero. Shorten the impulse say now 100 msec, again increase the intensity and note the current at which minimum accessible contraction is produced. Repeat this procedure by shortening the impulse duration say 30,10,3,1 and so on.

Drawing the Curve

After noting the current for various durations a graph is plotted with strength of current on Y axis and impulses or pulse durations on X axis.

Characteristics of Strength Duration Curves

It is the shape of curve, which is an important feature in determining the status of muscle innervations. So when all the nerve fibres supplying the muscles are intact then strength duration curve is typical like the Figure 4.1.

Normal Innervation

Strength duration curve with normal status of innervation of muscle will have various characteristics such as; initial portion of the

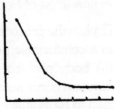

Fig. 4.1: Normal curve

graph is a straight line, which is parallel to the X axis, there is no kink, the graph is complete in other words it is plotted from highest duration such as 300 millisecond up to 0.01, rise in graph line occurs around 1msec duration. Graph looks smooth. The curve of this typical shape is there because equal strength of current is required to get minimum assessable response with longer durations while shorter pulses need a slight increase in the strength of stimulus each time when duration is shortened. The point at which this curve begins to rise is variable but usually it is 1millisecond with constant current.

Complete Denervation

The shape of the curve obtained on plotting of the strength duration curve of a muscle that is completely dene-ravated is typical in appearance. Initial part of the curve is not parallel. Plotted graph line look somewhat vertical line starting from the X axis. There is no kink in the curve. The graph line is incomplete because deneravted muscle does not

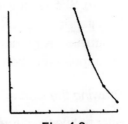

Fig. 4.2: Denervated curve

respond to smaller durations like 1, 0.3 0.1 and so on. This typical appearance is due to required increase in the strength of stimulus for all the impulses with a duration less than 100 millisecond. Response may not be obtained to very small durations and hence the curve rises steeply and is further to the right than that of a normally innervated muscle (Fig. 4.2).

Partial Denervation

The graph of a muscle that is partially innervated is typical in appearance. The plotted graph line shows kink. Kink appears because the graph shows the features of innervated as well as denervated muscle. It happens due to the response of the muscle to various impulses. Impulses with higher pulse durations stimulate denervated as well as innervated muscle fibers but the

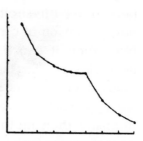

Fig. 4.3: Partial denervated curve

response to the smaller pulse durations is obtained by stimulating only innervated muscle fibers and hence to get minimal palpable or visible contractions from these innervated muscle fibers more intensity is required. Appearance of kink may give an approximate idea about the extent or proportion of innervation and denervation. If a large number of fibres are denervated then greater part of curve resembles to that of denervated muscles and vice versa. If the kink is located exactly at the center then one may conclude that innervation and denervation may be 50%. But if the three-fourth of the graph appears like innervated and one-fourth appears like denervated then innervation could be 75% and denervation could be 25%. Appearance of kink can have two interpretations. If initially muscle showed strength duration curve of complete denervation and later the appearance of kink that means that muscle is getting reinnervated. On the other hand a muscle initially showed normal strength duration curve and now kink that means this muscle is getting denervated. In progressive innervation or denervation the graph will move from the kink towards left side or right side respectively (Fig. 4.3).

Variations of Strength Duration Curve

Strength duration curve can be used to find out the status of sensory as well as motor nerve fibers. If we take into consideration only sensory threshold or current perception threshold (just perception of current) then it can be helpful in evaluating the status of A beta fibers, if we take motor level intensity then motor nerve fibers or A alpha and if we take suprasensory painful threshold then it can tell us the status of C fibers and A delta type of fibers. But hardly these variations are used clinically since there are sophisticated methods such as motor and sensory nerve conduction velocity tests which can be performed with electromyography. However, most commonly strength duration curve is used to find out motor nerve fiber innervation of muscles (Fig. 4.4).

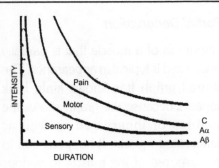

Fig. 4.4: Strength duration curve of sensory, motor and pain fibers

Advantages of Strength Duration Curve

Strength duration curve is simple, reliable and cheaper. It indicates proportion of denervation. It may be less time consuming as compared to electromyography. It can be used as hand side method.

Disadvantages of Strength Duration Curve

In large muscles only proportions of fibres may respond hence picture is not clearly shown. It's a qualitative rather than quantitative method of testing innervation. It won't point out the site of lesion. However, the site of lesion may be determined by nerve conduction test.

OTHER ELECTRODIAGNOSTIC TESTS

Pulse Ratio

Pulse ratio is the ratio of current needed to produce a muscle contraction with an impulse of 1millisecond to that of 100 milliseconds. In case of innervated muscle very small or no increase in current is required when impulse is reduced from 100 msec to 1msec. So the ratio is small and it is around 1 but it may vary up to 2.2 for innervated muscles (1:2.2). In case of denervated muscles amount of current required to produce a contraction is more and consequently the ratio is more than 2.5. Advantage of pulse ratio is, it can be performed swiftly. But the disadvantage is that the picture of innervation is not clear if a muscle is partially innervated.

Faradic IDC Test

It is also vaguely termed as faradic galvanic test rather than calling it as faradic interrupted direct current test. (Since galvanic current term indicates direct current and not modified direct or interrupted direct current). It was widely used in past to rule out whether a muscle is innervated or denervated. Pertaining to characteristics of faradic current (pulse duration 0.1 to 1msec and frequency 50 to 100Hz), it will stimulate only innervated muscles and not denervated muscles. Interrupted direct current with pulse duration such as 100 msec will stimulate both innervated and denervated muscles. If a muscle responds to interrupted direct current with 100msec duration or higher duration but not to faradic current then it may be a denervated muscle.

Nerve Conductivity Test

I personally prefer to call it as nerve transmission test in order to avoid the possibility of the confusion between nerve conductivity, nerve distribution and nerve conduction velocity tests. Normally a stimulus to a nerve trunk can produce the contractions of muscles supplied by it. But if the nerve fibers are degenerating then conductivity distal to the lesion is lost. For nerve conductivity test interrupted direct current with pulse duration of 0.1 or 0.3 millisecond is used. After applying this stimulus to a superficial nerve trunk, contractions of muscles supplied below this point is noted. If it produces the contractions then it suggests that at least few or all the nerve fibers are intact and functioning. If this test is performed along the course of a nerve then it may give us a clue about the possible site of the lesion.

Nerve Distribution Test

Stimulating the nerve trunk and observing the resultant muscle contractions can determine the distribution of nerve and thereby we can find out if there is any individual variation in it. This can help us to find out if there is any variation in the distribution of nerve.

Neurotization Time

Neurotization time is a useful index that represents the ratio of the duration of neuropathy to the theoretical time necessary for reinnervation to take place. In order to calculate the neurotization time measure the distance from the probable site of the lesion up to the distal most muscle supplied by the affected nerve in millimeter. Since the regeneration of nerve can occur at a rate of approximately one millimeter per day. Calculate the anticipated number of days accordingly (Remember that rate of nerve growth can vary from 1 to 5 mm per day). For instance if the distance of lesion is 105 mm then anticipated time is 105 days. Now find out the elapsed time in days from the patient. Calculate the neurotization time by following formula;

$$\text{Neurotization time} = \frac{\text{Elapsed time in days}}{\text{Anticipated time}} \times 100$$

Less than 100% neurotization time indicates that a minimal time is elapsed for reinnervation. When neurotization time is 250% or more and it is accompanied with no electrodiagnostic evidence of regeneration then the prognosis is poor and surgical inter-vention may be considered.

Galvanic Tetanus Ratio

Galvanic tetanus ratio (GTR) is also called as tetanic frequency ratio or the tetanus twitch ratio. Normally frequency of 20 to 50 cycles per second is required to get tetanic response with pulse duration equal to chronaxie but in case of denervated muscle it gets reduced to 5 to 10 cycles per second. This happens because of loss of accommodation to long durated impulses and slow type of contraction in denervated muscle. GTR requires the use of a stimulator with variable impulse frequency out put of 1 to 50 per second and calibrated duration of impulses. For testing deneravated muscle, this duration must correspond to the chronaxie. It is convenient, to stimulate the muscle with a single active electrode and with a current intensity sufficient to cause minimal contraction. Gradually vary the frequency, starting at a lower range like one per second until tetanus is produced.

Dermo-ohmometry

The study of human skin resistance is known as dermo-ohmometry. It may also be called as neurodermometry or galvanic skin response. It can be studied with GSR device that is at present rarely used for this purpose but it is now days used for relaxation purpose by incorporating it with biofeedback kind of devices. Normal skin resistance may vary from 10,000 to 20 million ohms depending on the distribution of the sweat glands. In complete lesion of a mixed nerve there is anhydrosis due to reduced activity of the sweat glands. As a result of anhydrosis there is increase in the skin resistance due to reduced sweat that permits easy passage of the current.

Polar Formula

It is also known as Erb's polar formula. Normal response obtained to cathode and anode is CCC>ACC>AOC>COC. Here CCC stands for cathodal closing current, ACC for anodal closing current, AOC for anodal opening current and COC for cathodal opening current. It means normally a better contraction is obtained with cathodal closing current than anodal closing current. Closing and opening terminologies are used because when this experiments must have been tried at that time simple key switch which is on by closing and off/by opening must have been used. In denervation reversal of this formula may be noted. In denervated muscle it may be ACC>CCC>AOC>COC.

Myotonic Reaction

In myotonic cases typical response to the faradic stimulation occurs. The muscles remain in tetanic contraction for some time as long as twenty seconds even after the stimulus has ceased. This response can be obtained initially and later on due to the exhaustion of the muscle contraction response ceases altogether but the same response once again can be obtained after a period of rest.

Reaction of Degeneration

Reaction of degeneration may occur following peripheral nerve injuries. Reaction of degeneration is of three types such as: complete reaction of degeneration (CRD), partial reaction of degeneration (PRD) and absolute reaction of degeneration (ARD).

Complete Reaction of Degeneration

Complete reaction of degeneration is also known as full or total reaction of degeneration. In complete reaction of degeneration, nerve does not respond to either faradic or interrupted galvanic current. However, muscle may respond to long durated pulse of interrupted galvanic current, muscle contraction is slow or sluggish, motor point may get shifted and polar formula may get reversed.

Partial Reaction of Degeneration

In partial reaction of degeneration there is decreased response by nerve to faradic and interrupted galvanic current. However, muscle may have decreased response to faradic but better response to interrupted galvanic current. The muscle contraction may be slow but it is not pronounced as in CRD.

Absolute Reaction of Degeneration

There is absence of any response to any current in muscle as well as nerve. It represents final stage of complete reaction of degeneration with unfavourable outcome. You should be sure of this before informing it to the patient.

ELECTROMYOGRAPHY

Definition

Electromyography is the study of electrical activity of muscle by means of surface electrodes placed over the skin or needle electrodes inserted in the muscle itself. By electromyography we can study motor unit potential, motor nerve conduction velocity, sensory nerve conduction velocity, etc. Electromyography is also called as electroneuromyography or ENMG. ENMG is a clinical electrophysiological evaluation, which consists of the observation, analysis and interpretation of the bioelectrical activity of muscle and nerve.

Uses

EMG is used to diagnose the diseases of muscle such as, myopathies, myasthenia gravis, etc. It can be used to differentiate between the lesions of anterior horn cells, the nerve fibres and the muscles. EMG can be used to determine sensory and motor nerves conduction velocities. EMG can be of major help in determining site, severity and prognosis of peripheral nerve lesions. EMG can analyze the muscle work involved in a complex activity.

Contraindications

Although electromyography with surface electrodes have very minimal contraindications, electromyography with needle electrodes is contraindicated in dermatitis, uncooperative patient, pacemaker, blood transmittable diseases, extreme swelling, abnormal blood clotting factor and patient on anticoagulant therapy. Gloves and eye protection should be used incase the EMG is to be done in individuals with blood transmittable diseases.

Equipment

Electromyography machine and various accessories consist of electrodes, preamplifier, amplifier, CRT display, stimulator, loudspeaker, and ancillary equipment (Fig. 4.5).

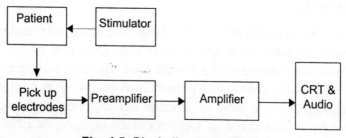

Fig. 4.5: Block diagram of EMG

Electrodes

Electrode is a device or metal conductor, which introduces or picks up electricity from the tissues. In other words electrode is a conductor that stimulates or record the electrical activity of tissues.

Stimulating electrode: In EMG study, electrodes are required to stimulate or evoke action potential in excitable tissues of interest that is muscle or nerve. Stimulating electrode is a bipolar hand held electrode that consists of anode and cathode separated by 2 to 3 cm distance. It is used to stimulate or activate peripheral nerve and or muscle during electrophysiological assessment.

Pick up electrodes: In order to monitor the responses of excitable tissues to voluntary or evoked potential, pick up electrodes are used. These pick up electrodes record the electrical activity from the tissues of interest. Pick up electrodes are active electrode, reference electrode and ground electrode (you can memorize them by RAG, where R stands for reference, A for active and G for ground). Active electrode is an electrode which actually pick up the potential difference from the tissues. Reference electrode is an electrode that helps to pick up potential difference by acting as a reference terminal, which completes the circuit. Ground electrode is an electrode, which is also known as zero potential electrode or shield electrode or guard electrode. It is made-up of metal and is usually larger than active and reference electrode. It is placed on the body surface at some distance over an area of little electrical activity such as bony prominences.

Active and reference electrodes are of two main types such as surface and needle electrodes.

Surface electrodes: Surface electrodes are placed on the skin to pick up the electrical activity. These are generally made-up of metals such as silver, gold, platinum. An efficient conduction through these electrodes can be obtained if skin is prepared by cotton swab dipped in spirit and by placing an electoconductive gel in between the electrodes and the skin. A surface electrode varies from 0.5 cm to several cm in diameter. These electrodes must be held firmly in place with adhesive tape or straps in order to obtain constant recording of electrical muscle activity.

These electrodes are used when the excitable tissues include a comparatively large area. Metal disc electrode, dual electrode, spring electrode are the commonly used types of surface electrode.

Needle electrodes: Needle electrodes are placed underneath the skin either near or directly in the excitable tissues of interest. They are prepared from platinum, silver or stainless steel. Needle electrodes are used when activity of very few motor units or muscle fibers is to be studied. This can be done easily with these electrodes as they have reasonably small exploring surface. Different types of needle electrodes are monopolar, concentric, bipolar, multielectrode, etc.

Preamplifier

It is a device, which increases the magnitude of potentials picked up by the electrodes so that they can be carried to the amplifier without getting influenced by unwanted potentials. It is usually situated in a remote box connected to the main EMG system by a cable on one side and on other side to the pickup electrodes through leads. This arrangement allows the preamplifier to be placed close to the electrodes to which it is directly connected by reasonably short leads in order to minimize the interference. Preamplifier reduces the noise as it amplifies the magnitude and the strength of pickup potentials. Noise is nothing but any interfering, unwanted interference. It may arise from internal or external source and hence noise can be termed as internal noise or external noise. Internal noise originates within the system. External noise originates from external sources such as electric wiring in the building, relay transmitters, radio frequency, etc. External noise is also known as interference or artifact. Preamplifier allows differential amplification by selecting amplification of original potentials while rejecting interfering potentials.

Amplifier

It follows preamplifier. It is an electronic machine, which is used to increase the amplitude of electrical signal level fed by preamplifier. Amplifier is used to make small electrical signals larger on signal display instrument such as oscilloscopes, computer screen or strip chart recorders. A characteristic feature of an amplifier is its gain. Gain is the relationship between input voltage amplitude of the signal and output voltage amplitude from the amplifier. If the peak voltage of a monophasic input signal is doubled from 2mV to 4mV then the gain of the amplification is 2 and if the same output signal's peak amplitude is increased to 10mV then the gain of amplification is 5. Most amplifiers are constructed so that the users can adjust the amplifier gain to a suitable level. The amplifier control for such adjustment is often labeled as sensitivity. Frequency response or filter control in amplifier responds to low and high frequency limits adjusted with frequency response controls in order to minimize noise. Amplifier may be a simple or differential amplifier. A simple amplifier is a device that enhances all voltage differences between recording electrodes. Differential amplifier is the amplifier, which increases the difference between the two signals. As biological potentials are generally of several orders and magnitude, lower amplitude than 60Hz interferes and the use of simple amplifier may not allow the examiner to adequately visualize the bioelectrical potentials of interest. To overcome this a differential amplifier is used. The differential amplification technique rejects signals that are common to both electrodes and enhances signals that are different. This is called common mode rejection. Differential amplifier uses a ground electrode to compare the signals of the two recording electrodes. Noise appears identical at both electrodes and will be rejected by common mode.

Cathode Ray Tube Display

EMG display or CRT display is used to visualize recorded action potentials in form of amplitude versus time graph. It consists of following parts, evacuated envelope, electron gun, horizontal deflection plates and vertical deflection plates.

Ancillary Equipment

For documentation, measurement and verification of transient potentials, an ancillary equipment records CRT display. Ancillary equipment may be an instant photographic camera, fiber optic recorder, digital storage time transformation recorders, magnetic recorders, etc.

Loud Speaker

A loud speaker is used in EMG apparatus so as to produce audible sounds for audio monitoring. These audible sounds are produced when recorded and amplified potentials are applied to speaker. It allows acoustic monitoring of the potentials.

MOTOR UNIT POTENTIALS

Various features of the normal motor unit potential are described here and before reading the same please refer the figure 4.6.

Normal Motor Unit Potential

Total Duration

It is the duration between initial deviations from the baseline to the return to the baseline. Total duration depends on the amplification gain, filter and whether or not the units are averaged. It varies between 5-10 ms.

Spike Duration

It is the time from the onset of the initial negative spike to the last most positive directed spike. It is 2 to 10 millisecond.

Amplitude

It is the maximum voltage measured from peak to peak. The density of muscle fibres, their diameters and how close together are their end plates or how synchronously they discharges determines amplitude. Amplitude varies greatly in normal muscles. It may be 100 to 200 microvolts.

Phases

Motor units are usually biphasic or triphasic. Biphasic when recorded at end plate. Triphasic when recorded away from end plate zone. The total number of phases is determined by adding one to the number of base line crosses. A MUP (motor unit potential) is considered polyphasic if it has greater than four phases. Frequently the MUPs have a saw

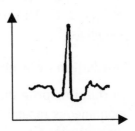

Fig. 4.6: Normal EMG

tooth like pattern where there are many changes of directions or turns but not actual baseline crosses. These potentials are referred to as serrated MUPs and are the measurements of the synchronicity of the muscle fibers discharging. Parameters of normal unit potential are amplitude: 100 to 200 μv (micro volt), duration: 2 to10 ms, waveform: 2 to 4 phases but usually triphasic, frequency: 1 to 60 per second (150 in eye muscles), sound: clear sharp thump or plunk and rise time: 100 to 200 seconds (Fig. 4.6).

Polyphasic Potential

The EMG examination may reveal complex shape than normal motor unit potentials. These are supposed to be the electrical expressions of a degenerating or regenerating but not denervated motor units. It arises from nonsynchronous firing of many muscle fibers comprising a motor unit. If this polyphasicity occurs in a muscle, which has previously demon-

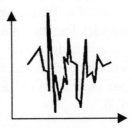

Fig. 4.7: Polyphasic potential

strated widespread fibrillation on potentials of denervation such polyphasics potentials are often called nascent motor units. Parameters of polyphasic potentials are amplitude: 20 to 5000 microvolts, duration: 2 to 25msec, waveform: 5 to 25 phases, frequency: 2 to 30 per seconds and sound: rough, rasping or rattling. 1 to 12% of normal EMG may show polyphasic potentials (Fig. 4.7).

Fibrillation Potential

Fibrillation potential occurs due to spontaneous repetitive contraction of a single muscle fiber. It is a fundamental sign of denervation. It appears in 15 to 20 days but do not appear immediately following nerve injury. It may occur as early as 5 days following nerve lesion. The fibrillation tracing always begins with a positive voltage. Parameters are,

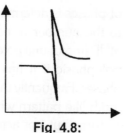

Fig. 4.8:
Fibrillation

amplitude: 10 to 600 microvolts, duration: 1 to 2 msec, waveform: mono or diphasic spike (usually diphasic), sound: sharp high-pitched click (like rain on the roof) (Fig. 4.8).

Positive Sharp Wave

It is found in denervation. It appears spontaneously, irregularly and is not predictable. It is seen in many denervated muscles. Parameters are, amplitude: very variable, duration: up to 100 msec, waveform: diphasic, frequency: 2 to 100 per second and sound: dull thud (Fig. 4.9).

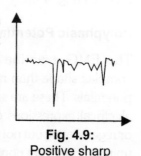

Fig. 4.9:
Positive sharp

Nerve Potential

It occurs when a needle electrode comes in contact with nerve fibrils inside muscle substance. Parameters are amplitude: 20 to

250 microvolts, duration: 1 to 4 msec, waveform: biphasic, frequency: 30 to 150 per sec and sound: machine gun and high pitched.

Myotonic Potentials

It is a high frequency fibrillation like discharge. It is heard as a diving airplane. These are a train of positive waves, which vary in frequency and amplitude (Fig. 4.10).

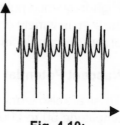

Fig. 4.10:
Myotonic

Fasciculation Potentials

It is spontaneously occurring potential over which the patient has no volitional control. It may be found in benign myokymia, anterior horn cell disease, nerve compression, various forms of muscle cramps, alkalotic states and incipient tetany.

They occur irregularly at a rate varying 1 to 50 per minute. They are of two types, simple and complex. Simple fasciculations are biphasic or triphasic and complex fasciculations are polyphasic. Polyphasic fasciculation potentials can be further divided into usual polyphasic fasciculation potential and iterative polyphasic potential on the number of isoelectric crosses (Fig. 4.11).

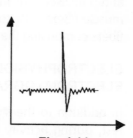

Fig. 4.11:
Fasciculation

Giant Potential

These are MUPs with more than 200 microvolts and duration 12 to15 milliseconds. They are frequently seen in anterior horn cell diseases like amyotrophic lateral sclerosis or poliomyelitis. It may be because of selective destruction of small motor units so that only the large ones are intact. It may be because of sprouting of the intact motor neuron branches to its denervated neighbors thus enlarging the scope of the neuron. Its stimulation firing will therefore give a giant potential.

Bizarre High Frequency Discharge

High frequency polyphasic discharges up to 200 per seconds are seen in variety of motor neuron diseases. It may be because of muscle spindle firing of atrophied muscle.

Nascent Potential

These are also termed as reinnervation potentials. They are low amplitude 50 to 200 mv, highly polyphasic that appear in the process of reinnervation. Initially they may appear involuntary and may be excited by tapping the muscle.

Myopathic Potentials

These are motor unit potentials with reduced amplitude and duration. Their amplitude varies from 50 to 200 μv in amplitude and 5 milliseconds in duration. They result from destruction of muscle fibers with consequent reduction in number of muscle fibers comprising the motor unit.

ELECTROPHYSIOLOGICAL TESTS WITH ELECTROMYOGRAPHY

In addition to the study of electrical activity of the muscle at rest, during activity and motor unit potential study, electro-myography can be used for other electrophysiological studies such as nerve conduction tests, blink reflex, evoked potentials, H reflex, F wave test, etc. Here I am just adding a brief idea about these tests since the more detailed technique of these tests is out of the scope of this book and can be studied from any other book revealing it.

Nerve Conduction Velocity

Nerve conduction velocity is an electrophysiological investigation by which velocity of propagation of impulses by a nerve is calculated. There are two types of nerve conduction velocities such as motor nerve conduction velocity and sensory nerve conduction velocity.

Blink Reflex Test

Blink reflex test is used to assess the functional integrity of both trigeminal and facial nerve. Blink reflex is used for identifying pathologies affecting cranial nerves such as Bell's palsy, cerebellar pontine angle tumors, Gullain Barre syndrome and central demyelinating diseases.

Central Evoked Potentials

These are voltage changes monitored from the tissues of cerebral cortex, brainstem and spinal cord in response to various applied sensory stimuli. Thus function of somatosensory cortex, visual cortex and auditory region of brainstem can be evaluated. They are of various types such as somatosensory evoked potentials (SSEP), brain stem auditory evoked potentials (BAEP), visual evoked potentials (VEP) and repetitive nerve stimulation (RNS or Jolly test).

H Reflex Test

It is also known as H wave or Hoffman response. It can be performed in upper and lower limb so as to get quantitative information about the stretch reflex pathway. In simpler words it is an electrically elicited monosynaptic reflex.

F Wave Test

It is an evoked response due to antidromically-propagated action potentials transmitted to the anterior horn cells or initial segment of alpha motor neuron axons. F wave test is used when the disease or injury is thought in the proximal segment of nerves for example nerve compression in thoracic outlet syndrome.

SUMMARY

Electrodiagnostic tests include rheobase, chronaxie, strength duration curve, pulse ratio, galvanic tetanic ratio, nerve conduction test, nerve distribution test, nerve conduction velocity, faradic galvanic test, etc. Strength duration curve is simple, reliable and cheaper form of elctrodiagnostic test. Following completed denervation reversal of polar formula may occur. Electromyography is the study of electrical activity of muscle by means of surface electrodes placed over the skin or needle electrodes inserted in the muscle itself. Normal EMG waveform is triphasic.

chapter five

Thermotherapy

SHORT WAVE DIATHERMY

Short wave diathermy is most commonly used physiotherapeutic modality for deep heating. The meaning of diathermy is heat given through an object and not confined to that object (Nagel Schmidt 1908). Short wave diathermy is used for more than fifty years by physiotherapists around the globe for deep heating purpose. For short wave diathermy, high frequency current with a frequency of 27.12 MHz and 11 meters wavelength is used. Other high frequency currents with their corresponding wavelengths, which are less commonly used, are 45 MHz with 7 metre and 13 MHz with 22 metre.

PRODUCTION

Principle

It is not possible to produce high frequency current required for short wave diathermy purpose by mechanical means. Hence, discharging a condenser through an inductance of low ohmic resistance produces the high frequency current with desired frequency and wavelength (Fig. 5.1).

Circuit

The basic circuit consists of two parts such as oscillator circuit and resonator circuit. In addition to this, an ammeter can be integrated in resonator circuit so as to register the resonance between oscillator circuit and resonance circuit.

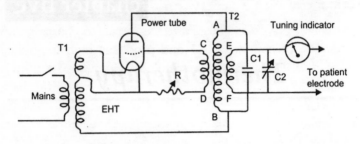

Fig. 5.1: Circuit diagram of short wave diathermy.
In figure, T1: step up transformer, T2: step down transformer, R: variable resistance, AB: inductance coil of oscillator circuit, ABC1 and power tube: oscillator circuit, CD: feedback coil which controls grid potential and EFC2: resonator circuit.

Oscillator Circuit

It consists of condenser and inductance. The values of condenser and inductance are such that they produce high frequency current with a frequency of 27.12 MHz. A valve is used along with condenser and inductance so as to allow repeated charging and discharging of the condenser.

Resonator Circuit

It is also known as patient's circuit. It consists of a variable condenser and an inductance coil. High frequency currents are transmitted from oscillator circuit to resonator circuit with the help of variable condenser.

Ammeter

The ammeter does not show the amount of current received by the patient but it show when the oscillator and resonating circuits are in tune with each other. In most of imported machines there is automatic tuner (just like television sets) and hence ammeter is not included in these types of machines.

Working

When mains are switched on, it causes repeated charging and discharging of condenser C1 and produces high frequency current in oscillator circuit. As a result high frequency current is also likely to develop in resonator circuit but maximum high frequency current can be produced in resonator circuit if oscillator and resonator circuit are in tune or resonance with each other. Tuning can be obtained manually by varying the capacity of C2 condenser and the same can be confirmed from ammeter, which will show maximum deflection if these two circuits are in resonance with each other. In automatic tuner the machine does this automatically. Output is controlled by power or intensity control of the machine, which regulates the output by adjusting the grid bias of valve through variable resistance.

ELECTRODES AND ARRANGEMENT OF ELECTRODES

Electrodes are conductors through which current is applied to the body tissue. In case of short wave diathermy, electrodes are the conductors through which short wave diathermy current is applied. Nowadays pad electrode, disc electrode, monode, minode, drum electrode and occasionally sinus electrodes are used for short wave diathermy applications. However, in past number of electrodes such as: cable electrode, axillary electrode, rectal electrode and vaginal electrode were used.

Condenser field electrodes such as pad or disc electrodes can be arranged in monopolar, coplanar, contra planar and cross fire arrangement. In monopolar arrangement one electrode that may act as an active electrode is placed over the area to be treated and other indifferent electrode is applied to some distant part of the body with maximum spacing so that the heating is produced at only the area treated. In coplanar arrangement, electrodes are placed side by side on the same aspect of the part to be treated, provided that there is an adequate distance between them. This arrangement is commonly used in the treatment of back. In contra planar arrangement, electrodes are placed over opposite aspects of the body part treated so that high frequency current is directed through the tissues. Contra planar method is commonly used in the treatment of hip joint. In cross fire arrangement half the treatment is given with the electrodes in one position then the arrangement is changed so that the electric field lies at right angles to the electric field obtained in the first part of treatment. It is commonly used in the treatment of knee joint, treatment of sinuses, pelvis and thorax.

While arranging the electrodes during the treatment consideration should be given to the size of electrode, electrode spacing and position of electrode. Size of electrode should be larger than the body part to be treated, spacing should be as wide as the output of machine permits and in the space between electrode and the body part there should be a medium with low dielectric constant such as air, felt with air columns or towels. Electrodes should be positioned in such a way that they are parallel to the body part to be treated.

PHYSIOLOGICAL EFFECTS

The main physiological effect of short wave diathermic current on the body tissue is heat production and other physiological effects results from the increase in temperature.

Temperature

Short wave diathermy application produces heat in the body tissues. Increase in local temperature may occur due to the production of heat. But if the short wave diathermy is applied for prolonged time then there is rise in general body temperature by few degrees. General rise in body temperature occurs due to blood that passes through the tissues in which the rise of temperature has occurred, it also becomes heated and carries heat to other parts of the body.

Metabolism

Metabolism is the collective process by which living status of tissues or the body is maintained. When short wave diathermy is applied to the body tissue then it produces heat. Heat production in the body tissues increases the metabolism. This may occur as per the Van't Hoff statement. Van't Hoff has stated that any chemical change capable of being accelerated by heat is accelerated by rise in temperature.

Blood Supply

Short wave diathermy application increases the local blood supply. Increase in blood supply may occur due to the direct effect of heat on the vessels in terms of vasodilatation. Vasodilatation may occur indirectly due to the action of metabolites on the vessel walls. Metabolites and other waste products production is increased due to increase in metabolic activity. Due to increased vasodilatation there is increase in the lumen of the vessels, which leads to increased blood supply.

Effect on Nerves

Mild heating due to short wave diathermy application may reduce the excitability of the nerves especially sensory nerves.

Muscle Relaxation

Rise in temperature induces relaxation of muscles and increase their efficacy of action. The muscle fibres contract and relax very easily but strength of the contraction is unaffected.

Tissue Damage

Excessive heating due to short wave diathermy application may cause the damage to the tissues in form of coagulation or thermal burns.

Blood Pressure

Prolonged application of short wave diathermy can reduce the blood pressure. This happens due to reduction in peripheral resistance to the flow of blood due to generalized vasodilatation and reduction in viscosity of the blood.

Sweating

Increase in the local and general temperature can cause increased sweating either in the local region of heating or generalized depending on the extent of heating.

THERAPEUTIC EFFECTS AND USES

Pain Relief

Short wave diathermy is one of the effective modality in relieving the musculoskeletal pain. Exact mechanism of pain relief is not known. But it may occur due to sedative effect of short wave diathermy on sensory nerves, counter irritation by heat, due to resolution in inflammation and due to the relief of underlying muscle spasm. However, in very acute conditions (less than 72 hours of onset) short wave diathermy application may increase the pain due to increase in the inflammatory process.

Muscle Spasm

Short wave diathermy can induce the muscle relaxation and hence, it can be used in the treatment of muscle spasm.

Joint Stiffness

Short wave diathermy can minimize the joint stiffness due to increased extensibility of connective tissue as a result of increase in local temperature and due to the relief of pain, spasm and inflammation. Usually short wave diathermy is used in the treatment of deep joint where superficial heating modalities may not be effective because of their smaller depth of penetration. In order to make use of this effect short wave diathermy should be applied prior to the manual therapy.

Inflammation

Increase in the blood supply increases white blood cells, antibodies and other essential nutritive materials. Increase in all of these may help in resolution of inflammation. Short wave diathermic application can minimize or resolve the subacute and chronic inflammation. It may resolve or minimize the acute inflammation provided it is applied at precise time following the onset of acute inflammation (after 72 hours) with right dosages otherwise it can aggravate the acute inflammatory process.

Musculoskeletal Trauma

Short wave diathermy accelerates the healing by increasing the amount of nutritive materials required for healing following musculoskeletal trauma.

INDICATIONS AND CONTRAINDICATIONS

Indications

Short wave diathermy can be used in the treatment of various orthopedic as well as some of non-orthopedic conditions.

Orthopedic conditions low back pain, osteoarthritis, rheumatoid arthritis, sprains, strains, muscle tear, tendon tear, capsulitis, tendonitis, frozen shoulder, mayalgia, bursitis, hematoma, neuralgia, neuritis, traumatic arthritis, ankylosing spondylitis, fibrositis, etc.

Sports Injuries rectus femoris strain, hamstrings strain, tensor fascia lata strain, hip pointer and contusions to thorax.

Surgical conditions infected surgical incisions and stitch abscess.

ENT conditions chronic sinusitis and chronic otitis media.

Chest conditions chronic bronchitis, chronic obstructive airway disease, pleurisy and pleuritis.

Gynecological conditions nonspecific pelvic inflammatory disease.

Other conditions abscess, inflammation of gallbladder and ducts, peritoneal adhesions and prostatitis.

Contraindications

Short wave diathermy is contraindicated in presence of pregnancy, cardiac pace maker, hemorrhage, thrombosis, peripheral vascular diseases, metal implants, impaired sensations, anesthetic areas, malignancy, following X-ray therapy, epileptic patients, mentally retarded patients, patients who are unable to communicate and fever.

Precautions

Precaution should be taken while treating patients with hearing aids, contact lenses and electrophysiological orthoses. Contact lenses should be removed for the treatment in the vicinity of head neck face region. Electrophysiological orthoses and hearing aid can be switched off or removed during the treatment. It is also important to keep the transistorized units such as TENS units, muscle stimulators, phones, mobiles, electronic calculators, electronic watches, interferential therapy unit and electronic traction devices at least 5 to 10 feet away from the short wave diathermy machine.

Dosages of Short Wave Diathermy

In acute conditions short wave diathermy is applied for 5 to 10 minutes once or twice daily and in chronic conditions it is applied for 20 to 30 minutes. Intensity should be chosen in such a way that it produce mild comfortable and perceptible warmth. In another words it should raise the temperature of the tissues to safer therapeutic range, which is 40 to 45 °C. In the past the dosages were chosen from four levels. Level I: unnoticeable heat, level II: slightly noticeable heat, level III: more noticeable heat and level IV: very noticeable heat.

Advantages of Short Wave Diathermy

Heat is produced in the body tissue and not transmitted through the skin, localization of heat can be done by careful placement of electrodes, deep heating is possible, there is no discomfort to the patient as high frequency current of short wave diathermy do not stimulate sensory and motor nerves and treatment can be controlled precisely.

PULSED SHORT WAVE DIATHERMY

In pulsed mode of short wave diathermy the output of high frequency current commences and ceases at regular interval. In other words, the output is applied in form of series of short bursts. Pulsed short wave diathermy is also called as pulsed electromagnetic energy, pulsed peak power, diapulse, etc. In 1930s pulsed short wave diathermy was invented but it became popular after 1950. Pulsed short wave diathermy produces non-thermal effects mainly. As a result there is no appreciable heat developed during the treatment. Pulsed short wave diathermy increases the cellular activity, increases reabsorption of hematoma, reduces inflammation, reduces swelling and increases the repair process. Various parameters of pulsed short wave diathermy include pulse duration, pulse repetition, intensity or pulsed peak power, mean power, etc. The treatment duration of pulsed short wave diathermy ranges from 15 to 60 minutes and the indications and contraindications are more or less same as that of continuous short wave diathermy.

MICROWAVE DIATHERMY

Microwave diathermy can be defined as the therapeutic use of the microwaves for the treatment of various diseases and disorders. Microwave diathermy is also called as microthermy. Microwaves are electromagnetic waves with wavelength in between 1 cm and 1 meter. For physiotherapeutic purpose high frequency current of 2450 MHz and wavelength 12.25 cm or 433.92 MHz and 69 cm are used. Considering the electromagnetic spectrum, one can very well note that the wavelength of microwaves lies between infra red and short waves.

PRODUCTION

Principle

It is not possible to produce microwaves by mechanical means and hence they are produced from magnetron, which is a special type of thermionic valve.

Functional Parts

Microwave diathermy apparatus consists of following functional parts; power supply, magnetron oscillator circuit, magnetron oscillator, intensity control, coaxial cable and emitter. Power supply supplies high voltage pulsed direct current and magnetron oscillator circuit control adequate heating and cooling of magnetron. The primary function of magnetron oscillator is to produce high frequency current required for the production of microwaves. Magnetron is a special type of thermionic valve characterized by centrally placed cathode, which is surrounded by circular type metal anode. Anode has circular cavities that allow the production of circulating or alternating current. Coaxial cable carries the high frequency currents from magnetron and fed it to the antenna of the emitter. Emitter is also known as director or applicator. Emitter consists of antenna and reflector. Antenna is mounted in front of a metal reflector. Reflector is metal plate, which directs the waves in only one direction. Emitters are available in various sizes and shapes. Emitter can be kept in contact with the body if there is internal spacing in it, otherwise it should be kept at a distance of 10 to 20 cm from the body surface to be treated. Intensity knob controls the output of the microwave by varying the power supplied to the magnetron (Fig. 5.2).

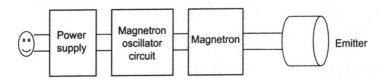

Fig. 5.2: Block diagram of microwave diathermy

Physiological and Therapeutic Effects

Physiological and therapeutic effects of the microwave diathermy are same as that of the short wave diathermy. But the amount of heat production is more in muscles as compared to short wave diathermy since the heat production by the microwaves depends on the watery content of the tissues. The depth of penetration of microwaves is smaller and ranges in between 3 mm to 3 cm while in case of short wave diathermy it may be up to 6 cm.

Uses and Contraindications

Uses of the microwave diathermy are same as that of short wave diathermy. Degenerative arthropathy, enthesopathies, chronic pleurisy, chronic bronchitis, chronic sinusitis, chronic adenitis, mastitis, mammary abscess, boils, carbuncles, severe vaginal diseases, severe rectal diseases, diseases of the ear and arthritis of small joints can be treated by microwave diathermy.

Various contraindications to microwave diathermy applications are patients with cochlear implants, patients with metallic endoprosthesis in the area to be treated, patients with malignant tumors, patients with tuberculosis, patients with thrombosis, ischemia, varicose veins, necrosis, diminished or loss of thermal sensation, recent haemorrhage, and acute inflammation. Microwaves should not be applied into the region of eyes and testes.

Precautions should be taken while treating patients with an increased temperature, osteoporotic patients, pregnant women, patients with intrauterine contraceptives and the application in the area of the lower abdomen during menstruation in females.

Dosages of Microwave Diathermy

Dosages of microwave diathermy are, in acute conditions 5 to 10 minutes and in chronic conditions 20 to 30 minutes with an output, which will produce just perceptible and comfortable warmth. It can be measured and up to 200 watts can be given so as to raise the body tissue temperature in therapeutic range of 40 to 45°C.

Oudin Current

Oudin current is rarely used now days due to the recognition of short wave diathermy by most of the physiotherapists around the world. In general, it is monoterminal high frequency current in the range of long wave band. It is often marketed as Heal-O-Ray or just by the name high frequency unit. It fascinates me as well as my patients. I may prefer this current sometimes in those patients who do not respond to other forms of treatments. These patients like the sparkling sound that occurs during the treatment and the pinkish color in the glass electrode. This current is applied through the glass vacuum electrode. In administering this current the glass electrode is held close to the body part to be treated. When the current is applied through the electrode it produces sparking. This produces counter irritation and hyperemia. This current may be considered in neuralgias, sprains, strains, myositis and sluggish noninfected wounds and ulcers. One should use this modality with caution, since the literature about the treatment parameters is not readily available and if applied with high intensity, high frequency and with very close proximity to the body part it can produce electrodessication.

PARAFFIN WAX BATH THERAPY

Treatment of various body parts with melted paraffin wax, whose temperature is maintained at 40 to 44°C, is known as paraffin wax bath therapy. The actual melting point of wax is 51 to 54.4°C. If this melted wax is poured directly on the body tissue then it may cause thermal injuries and hence to avoid this, melting point of wax is lowered by an addition of an impurity in form of paraffin oil. The heat transfer during paraffin wax bath therapy occurs through conduction from the layer of solid paraffin wax into the skin.

Paraffin Bath Unit

Parts of typical paraffin wax bath unit used in hospital setups are container, mains, thermostat, thermostat pilot lamp, cap and casters. Container is made-up of steel. It contains wax and paraffin oil in 6:1 or 7:1 ratio. This ratio is used so that mixture will stay liquid at the applied temperature. Its function is to maintain wax in melted status. Function of mains is to switch on or off the heating element, which is located in the casing of paraffin wax bath unit. Power pilot's function is to show whether power is on or off. Thermostat pilot's lamp indicates whether thermostat is on or off. Thermostat keeps the temperature fixed or static in the range, which is adjusted with knob. Cap covers the container when it is not in use and casters allow the paraffin wax bath container to be moved from one place to another.

Clinical Effects and Uses of Paraffin Wax Bath Therapy

Paraffin wax bath can relieve musculoskeletal pain, reduce stiffness, increase the local temperature, increase sweating, increase the local circulation and increase the pliability of skin. Clinically paraffin wax bath therapy is used in the treatment of osteoarthritis, rheumatoid arthritis, tenosynovitis, joint stiffness, leprosy, scleroderma, Dupytren's contracture, Sudeck's atrophy and various soft tissue contractures.

Contraindications

Paraffin wax bath therapy is contraindicated in presence of open wounds, since it may enter in the wound and act as a foreign body and delay healing. Infective conditions should not be treated by paraffin wax bath as it may increase inflammatory process. Allergic rashes, deep vein thrombosis, impaired sensations and skin conditions like acute dermatitis should not be treated with paraffin wax bath therapy.

METHODS OF APPLICATION

Dip Method

It provides mild heating. The patient should wash and dry the part to be treated. The therapist instruct the patient to dip the body part in the bath and then remove it until the paraffin solidifies and a thin layer of adherent solid paraffin is formed which covers the skin. Dipping is repeated until a thick coat is formed. In other words at least 8 to 12 times until the wax has formed a thick glove over the part. Once the thick glove of wax is formed, the treated area should be wrapped first in plastic and then over wrapped with towel. If oedema is a concern then the area may be elevated. The effective duration of this treatment is 10 to 15 minutes. At the end of this treatment time the glove of solid wax is peeled off or removed by slipping a finger beneath the glove and sliding the wax off and into the plastic sack, which covered it during the treatment. The sack is then discarded or the wax is emptied into the bath unit.

Immersion Method

This method of application provides somewhat vigorous heating. The body part to be treated is dipped 3 to 4 times to form a thin coat and then left immersed in paraffin for 20-30 minutes. A thin glove of solid paraffin wax forms slows the heat conduction. Use of the immersion method requires co-operation and tolerance by the patient in a dependent position. Care should be taken to ensure that the patient is in comfortable position during the treatment. With immersion method the temperature elevation of the body tissue is 2°C higher than dipping method.

Brush Method

It is a less commonly used method of paraffin wax application. In this method, 8 to 10 coats of wax are applied to the area with a paintbrush using even and rapid strokes. The area is then wrapped with towels for 10 to 20 minutes and after this time paraffin wax is removed and discarded.

Bandage Method

In this method, bandage of a suitable size and mesh is soaked in hot wax and then it is wrapped around the limb. Additional wax then can be poured or brushed over the bandage.

Technique of Application

Explain the procedure, expose the body part to be treated, remove the jewelry, check the sensation, check for contra-indications, inspect the body part to be treated before, ensure the comfortable position of the patient, check the temperature selected on thermostat before treatment, double check or recheck by inserting finger into the bath, use any method of application which is convenient for you and your patient, and apply paraffin wax, inspect the body part treated after the treatment.

Maintenance of Paraffin Wax Bath Unit

Sterilize the paraffin wax bath by heating it to 212° Fahrenheit or as directed by the manufacturer. For reuse sterilization should be done frequently. Drain the melted paraffin wax, filter it out and replace it back for reuse. Change the wax at least once in six months.

HOT PACKS

Hot pack is one of the superficial heating agents used for thermotherapy. They are used to alleviate muscle spasm, increase range of movement and for pain relief. However, hot packs should not be used in an area of impaired sensation, recent haemorrhage, open wounds and impaired circulation.

Physiological and Therapeutic Effects

Local Temperature

Rise in local body temperature occurs following hot packs application. It is due to the conduction of heat from hot pack to the skin and superficial tissues. The increase of body temperature is expected to be less than 45°C otherwise tissue burn will occur. This rise of temperature is proportional to the area of tissue exposed and the temperature of the hot pack.

Circulation

Increase in tissue temperature is associated with vasodilatation. As a result of vasodilatation local increase in the blood supply especially in the superficial tissue is likely to occur. It may be manifested by hyperemia. Vasodilatation may be due to release of chemical mediators, local spinal cord reflex and cutaneous thermoreceptor.

Pain Relief

Hot packs can be used to obtain analgesia. Pain relief following hot pack application may occur due to decreased nerve conduction velocity or elevated pain threshold. It may be due to sedative or counter irritation effect by heat. Pain relief may occur due to relief of muscle spasm if pain is associated with muscle spasm.

Muscle Spasm

Hot pack can bring about the relief of muscle spasm but exact mechanism is unknown. It may be due to decreased alpha motor neuron firing as a result of reduced muscle spindle activity.

Connective Tissue Extensibility

Hot pack may increase the extensibility of connective tissues. It is due to the effect of heat on the elastic tissues. This effect is more if it is combined with the stretching.

TYPES OF HOT PACKS

Hydrocollator Packs

Hydrocollator packs provide superficial moist heat. The commercial hot packs consist of canvas bags. These bags are filled with silicate gel or some other hydrophilic substance. They are stored in a thermostatically controlled water bath inside equipment. Inside the bath it absorbs the water with its high heat content. Hydrocollator packs are available in variety of sizes and shapes and should be chosen on the basis of size and contours of the body part to be treated. The temperature of packs when applied should be in between 70 to75°C so that it raises the body tissue temperature to 40 to 45°C during the treatment period. *Technique:* Explain the procedure to the patient, expose the body part to be treated and check the thermal sensation (remember with SEE, S for sensation, E for expose and E for explanation). Position the patient. Lift the hydrocollator pack with scissor forceps from the hot pack machine. Wrap it in dry terry towel; usually 6 to 8 layers of towel are used in order to wrap the hydrocollator pack. Place the pack wrapped in towel over the area of treatment so that it will cover the treatment area adequately. Don't secure it tightly so that patient can remove it, if it becomes too hot. Ask the patient about sensation, it should be mild and perceptible warmth and discard the patient's feeling ' hotter the better '. Continue the treatment for 20 minutes and adjust the dosiometry by varying the thickness of the terry towel which intern slow down the heat transfer. If patient feels too hot then increase the toweling layer or remove the hydrocollator pack. Advice not to lie with body weight on the hydrocollator pack since it may squeeze the water; decrease circulation and there by the dissipation of the heat. Advantages of hot packs are; ease of application, it offers comfortable heat and it is relatively inexpensive from purchase and maintenance point of view. However, the disadvantages of hot packs are there is no temperature control once applied to the patient. It is sometimes awkward to secure in place on a patient. Hot packs do not retain heat longer than 20 minutes, it is a passive form of the treatment and do not require any active participation by the patient.

Hot Water Bag

The rubber bags containing hot water can be used in the same fashion as like hydrocollator packs. Usually hot water bags are advised for the home treatment.

Kenny Packs

These packs are named after Sister Kenny. Kenny pack consists of a woolen cloth, which is steered and then surplus water content is removed by spinning. The relatively dry pack is then applied quickly to the skin. It is usually applied at a temperature of 60°C. As it contains little water, it has got small heat carrying capacity and the temperature drops down suddenly to normal level in 5 minutes. It is a short term but vigorous heating application, which produces a marked reflex response.

Chemical Hot Packs

These chemical hot packs are recently available for therapeutic applications. The chemical hot packs are portable. These packs are flexible container bag like structures in which by moving the container a compartment is broken, this allows ingredient to get mixed or come together and produce elevation of temperature by exothermic reaction. All these packs are poorly controlled. Ingredients are irritating or harmful when outer pack breaks and content comes in contact with the skin. Hence this type of application is least advantageous.

Electrical Heating Pads

Electrical heating pad is a form of superficial heating agent. It can be advised to the patients for their home treatment. The advantages of electrical heating pads are; they are cheaper, flexible, patient can control the heat during the treatment through a knob and they provide comfortable heat. However, the patient should remain awake during the treatment with the electrical heating pad as there is a possibility that patient may sleep during the treatment and will get up to find the thermal burn. The temperature elevation occurs through the conduction of the heat from the heating pad to the body tissues where the electrical heating pad is applied. This can be used as an adjunct to the diathermy specially when diathermy machine goes out of order! or for home visits.

SUMMARY

Short wave diathermy is most commonly used physiotherapeutic modality for deep heating. Advantage of short wave diathermy is that the heat is produced in the body tissue and not transmitted through the skin. Pulsed short wave diathermy produces non-thermal effects mainly. Physiological effects, therapeutic effects and uses of the microwave diathermy are same as that of the short wave diathermy. Precautions should be taken while treating patients with an increased temperature, osteoporotic patients, pregnant women, patients with intrauterine contraceptives and female patient in the area of the lower abdomen during menstruation. Oudin current is used rarely and when applied through the glass electrode it produces sparking. The heat transfer during paraffin wax bath therapy occurs through conduction from the layer of solid paraffin wax into the skin. Infective conditions should not be treated by paraffin wax bath as it may increase inflammatory process. Hot pack is one of the superficial heating agents and increases the local temperature on its application. Electrical heating pads are cheaper, flexible and can be used by the patient at home.

chapter six

Therapeutic Ultrasound

INTRODUCTION

We can hear some one when he is talking to us. You can also hear melodious music from a stereo and if you like then you can hear the beating of a drum. It's possible for us to hear all these things because of the sound waves, which vibrates the matter and produces the sound. You can very well hear sound waves but cannot see them. We human beings hear the sound waves by our ears but there is limit for this. The limit is in form of frequency, we can hear the sound waves with a frequency of less than 20 KHz. The dictionary meaning of the word ultra is beyond. Since the ultrasound waves are beyond the audible capacity of the human ear, it justifies the name ultrasound instead of sound. Ultrasound can be defined as a form of acoustic vibrations occurring at a frequency that is too high to be perceived by the human ear. For the physiotherapeutic purpose ultrasound with a frequency in the range of 0.5 to 5 MHz is used. Most commonly 1 MHz frequency is used all over the world for physiotherapy purpose but in few countries even 3 MHz is commonly used. In ultrasound treatment stream of the pressure waves are transmitted to a small volume of tissue, which causes the molecules of the tissues to vibrate. Mechanical pressure wave of ultrasound is applied to the tissues at a level of intensity that is so low and at a frequency that is so rapid that the person receiving it cannot detect the pressure itself. Historically in 1920's ultrasound had been used for under water detection. However, then it was observed that extreme pressure waves were damaging to the living tissues. This lead to the first use of ultrasound in medicine, for the treatment of the cancer. During 1930's lower intensities of ultrasound were used for the first time in physical medicine to treat soft tissue conditions with mild heating. Ultrasonic therapy is better treatment than most of the other electrotherapeutic treatments because of its effective depth of penetration. Hence, ultrasound is one of the commonly used physiotherapeutic modality.

PRODUCTION

Principle of Production

It is not possible to produce ultrasound waves by mechanical means and hence, they are produced by the application of rapidly alternating current to the crystal of piezoelectric substances. For this purpose crystal of quartz, barium titnate, lead zirconate, germanium, etc can be used. These crystals can produce the ultrasonic waves on the basis of reverse piezoelectric effect. In 1888 Pierrie and Currie described the piezoelectric effect. The meaning of the word piezo is pressure. Application of pressure, compression or deformation to the crystal produces the electric changes in the crystal. In 1910 Langevin described the reverse piezoelectric effect. Reverse piezoelectric effect is the application of electricity or potential difference across the crystal produces oscillations or deformation or pressure changes in the crystal. From the ultrasonic point of view, the reverse piezo-electric effect is the production of high frequency oscillations from the crystal of piezoelectric substances by the application of high frequency current. (Memory trick: HFO of crystal by HFC).

Functional Parts

The functional parts of the ultrasonic generator are oscillator circuit, controlling circuit, resistance circuit, coaxial cable, crystal and transducer. Oscillator circuit produces high frequency alternating current, resistance circuit controls the amplitude of the ultrasound waves by controlling the amplitude of high frequency alternating currents and controlling circuit produces the pulsed out put. In addition to this there is a coaxial cable, which transfer the high frequency current from the generator to the crystal. Crystal acts as the source of ultrasound waves. Transducer or the head serves as an applicator.

Parameters

Various controlling knobs or the parameters of ultrasound machine are mains, timer, intensity or output, meter, space ratio, etc. The function of mains is to switch on or off the machine, the function of timer is to adjust the treatment time, the function of output knob is to adjust the intensity of sound waves, the meter helps to measure the dose, space ratio can be adjusted as per the requirement, usually higher output and less interval is preferred in chronic and reverse in case of acute. Hence in short, we can summaries it as 1:1 for chronic and 1:4 for acute and so on.

Working

When power is supplied to the circuit then oscillator circuit produces the high frequency circuit. Pulse mode switches on the controlling circuit and produces interrupted or pulsed out put. The power or output is then controlled by means of the resistance circuit.

The high frequency current produced by the generator is fed to the crystal via coaxial cable. It is applied by means of metal electrodes on either side of the crystal say top and bottom of it. Application of the high frequency current causes repeated oscillations of crystal with a high frequency and produces the ultrasound waves. On the front side of the crystal, metal plate or the diaphragm of transducer is located and on the backside of it, there is air column. The air column on the backside causes the emission of ultrasonic waves mostly from the front side or the treatment aspect of the transducer (Fig. 6.1).

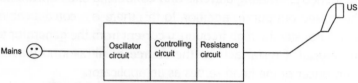

Fig. 6.1: Block diagram of ultrasonic generator

PHYSIOLOGICAL EFFECTS

Thermal Effects

When ultrasound waves are applied to the body tissues then tissues absorb them. As a result of absorption of ultrasound waves, heat is produced inside the body tissue. This heat may be produced because of the conversion of the sonic energy into the thermal energy. If heat dissipation equals the generation then there is no net rise in the local temperature and the effect is said to be non-thermal. On the other hand if heat dissipation is less than the generation then there is net rise in the local temperature and the effect is said to be thermal. Various thermal effects are increased peripheral arterial blood flow, increased tissue metabolism, increased permeability of membrane, increased pain threshold, increased sensitivity of C-type of nerve fibers, relief of muscle spasm, increased vascularity of skin due to stimulation of sympathetic fibers, increased tendon extensibility and may produce pathological fractures in bone with excessive dosages. It is also said that ultrasound may not have any beneficial effect on fracture healing.

The amount of the heat produced due to insonation depends on various factors such as intensity, mode, duration of insonation, space ratio, reflection of sound waves inside the tissues, protein content, etc. If the intensity is higher then there is more heat production. If the duration of insonation or ultrasound application is higher then there is more heat production inside the body tissues. If there is more reflection of the ultrasound waves inside the body tissues then there is more rise in local heat. Tissues with higher protein content absorb more ultrasound and hence, there is more production of heat if the protein content of the tissues is higher. The amount of the heat developed is more in continuous mode as compared to the pulsed mode. In case of pulsed mode it depends on space ratio and the heat production is more if space ratio is 1:1 than when it is 1:4 or 1:7. Heat produced is likely to be better if reflection is greater as a result of adding effect of propagation and reflected back waves. It occurs at interfaces of periosteum and bone, which are separated by a thin layer of air. As a result of reflection localized overheating at periosteum level may occur and may lead to periosteal pain or hot spots and hence during the treatment subcutaneous bony prominences may be avoided. Heating effect is also likely to be increased because of friction between ultrasound head and body tissue, non-moving ultrasound head, if ultrasound is used continuously, repeatedly without allowing sufficient time to cool off the ultrasound machine.

Thermal effect increases vasodilatation, cell activity, blood supply and removes waste products and there by facilitates resolution of inflammation and promotes healing. The thermal effect also causes increase in extensibility of fibrous tissues such as ligaments, joint capsule and scar tissues.

Mechanical Effects

Mechanical or non-thermal effects of therapeutic ultrasound are acoustic streaming, micromassage, standing waves and cavitations.

Acoustic streaming   Unidirectional flow of tissue fluids as a result of insonation is termed as acoustic streaming. Acoustic streaming increases permeability of cells.

Micromassage   Acoustic vibrations due to insonation produce a form of micro massage effect in the tissues.

Standing waves   Stationary or standing waves pattern of ultrasonic waves may develop if there is cancellation effect of propagating and reflected waves. Standing waves may produce blood cell stasis in the vessels and hence measures like moving the ultrasound head during the treatment or using pulsed form, etc should be taken so as to prevent the formation of standing waves pattern in the body tissues.

Cavitations   It is the formation of tiny gas bubbles in the tissues as a result of insonation. The size of these gas bubbles is of a micron. Cavitations may be stable or transient. In stable cavitations gas bubbles remains intact, size of bubbles does not change and there is no considerable pressure and temperature change. On the contrary in case of transient cavitations there is rapid change in the volume of bubbles. Collapsing of these bubbles causes considerable pressure and temperature changes and hence transient cavitations can cause gross damage to the tissues. To prevent the occurrence of cavitations adequate pressure with transducer should be exerted during the application, pulsed out put can be used, only suggested levels of insonation should be used and any sort of discomfort to the patient should be avoided during the treatment.

Chemical Effects

Insonation enhances chemical reactions and processes occurring at tissue level. The effect may be similar to a test tube shake in the laboratory.

THERAPEUTIC EFFECTS

Therapeutic effects of insonation are pain relief, resolution of inflammation and acceleration of healing.

Pain Relief

Pain can be relived by ultrasonic therapy. Insonation can be used for the relief of acute, subacute and chronic musculoskeletal pain. Exactly how it causes pain relief is not known. It may due to thermal or non-thermal effects. Pain relief may occur due to resolution of inflammation, removal of waste products or altered permeability of cell membrane to sodium, which may alter the electrical activity or pain threshold.

Inflammation

Insonation helps in the resolution of inflammation by increased blood supply, white blood cells and removal of waste products. Hence, it can be used in the treatment of inflammatory conditions and traumatic conditions to reduce the inflammation and prevent adhesions of soft tissues.

Effect on Healing/Repair

Healing may occur by repair or regeneration. Repair is the replacement of damaged cells by some other cells, which are not exactly similar in structure and function. Regeneration is the replacement of damaged cells by the same cells, which are same in structure and function. Human beings have lost their power of regeneration during evolutionary process and very little regeneration occurs in human beings. Ultrasound facilitates the healing at all three stages of repair. During inflammatory phase insonation increases the fragility of lysosomes. As a result there is release of autotytic enzymes. Autotytic enzymes clear the debris. In proliferative phase ultrasound increases the proliferation of fibroblasts and myofibroblasts. Myofibroblasts are the cells, which contain fibril like structure. In remodeling phase ultrasound facilitates remodeling of new tissues.

Therapeutic Uses

Therapeutic ultrasound has been applied to vast range of conditions. Few of conditions in which successful out come is likely to occur are; bursitis, tendonitis, plantar fascitis, plantar warts, calcaneal spur, tennis elbow, golfer's elbow, sacroilitis, coccydynia, low back pain, osteoarthritis, rheumatoid arthritis, fibrous nodules, rheumatic nodules, venous ulcers, scars, pressure sores, Dupuytren's contracture, later stages of myositis ossificans, phantom limb pain, frozen shoulder, temporo-mandibular joint syndrome, Bell's palsy, sports injuries, surgical wounds, episiotomies, capsulitis, joint contractures, deep seated muscle spasm, calcific tendonitis, exostosis, causalgia, Sudeck's atrophy, pyerione's disease, dislocations, sprains, etc.

Contraindications

Therapeutic ultrasound is contraindicated over metal implants, plastic implants such as high-density polyethylene, acrylic implant and implanted cardiac pace makers. Insonation over these implants may be harmful because of maximum absorption of acoustic vibrations, increased heat production and interference with the function of implants. Insonation is also contraindicated over specialized tissues such as eyes, ears, ovaries or testes as it may have harmful effects such as cavitations and may lead to irreparable damage.

An area where there is presence of vascular problems such as haemorrhage, haematoma, haemarthrosis, haemophilia, thrombosis, thrombophlebitis, embolism, arteriosclerosis and ischemia should not be treated with ultrasound. Insonation should not be applied in infected area, as there is possibility of spread of infection to the deeper level or to other patient through cross contamination. In tuberculous lesion it may reactivate the dormant capsular lesion. High doses of ultrasound should not be given over anesthetic areas so as to avoid possible skin damage because of heat. Ultrasound should not be applied to areas that have received radiotherapy within last six months as it may cause more devitalization of the tissues. Ultrasound therapy over tumor/neoplasm should be avoided as it may cause metastases. Treatment over or near the abdomen of pregnant patient with ultrasound should be avoided because it may produce untoward effects. Ultrasound therapy over spina bifida is generally avoided as it may have an adverse effect on spinal cord. Similarly, treatment over cervical ganglia or over vagus nerve is dangerous in patients who suffer from cardiac diseases.

Dangers and Precautions

Various dangers like thermal burns, cavitations, over dose, damage to the ultrasound machine, etc. is likely to occur during insonation. However, these dangers can be minimized or prevented by taking some precautions. Various precautions to be taken while treating a patient are; check the thermal sensation prior to the ultrasound application, use the suggested levels of ultrasound dosages, move the ultrasound head, avoid superficial bony prominences, avoid excess sensation of heat during the treatment, don't keep the ultrasound head in air when the output is on, maintain the perfect contact in between the ultrasound head and the body tissues, etc.

Methods of Application

Various methods by which insonation can be applied are bath method, bag method and through contact cream. (You can remember them with BBC).

Contact Cream Method

This method of ultrasound application is quite commonly used. It is also vaguely called as direct method. However, ultrasound cannot be applied directly to the body part since there are chances of reflections of ultrasound and uneven transmission without couplant. Couplant is any intervening material medium between ultrasound head and body tissue which offers perfect contact of head to the body tissue and allow maximum transmission of sonic waves. Various ultrasonic couplants used are boiled or degassed water, glycerin, oils, liquid paraffin and various ultrasonic gels commercially available for this purpose. Commercially available ultrasonic gels are thixotrophic in nature that is they liquefy very easily. In addition to this they are attractive in color, less corrosive to the skin, allow perfect contact between the ultrasonic head and the body tissues, allow satisfactory transmission, they can be easily wiped out and somewhat cheaper also!

In contact cream or the direct method coupling material such as ultrasonic gel is applied to the skin and the ultrasound head is moved over the area to be treated. This method is satisfactory for even body surfaces. During inso-nation with this method ultrasonic head should be kept in perfect contact with body tissues, head should be kept at right angle to the body surface treated and adequate pressure should be exerted (Fig. 6.2).

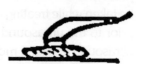

Fig. 6.2: Through contact cream

Insonation by Bath Method

It is also known as subacqeous method of application. In bath method, insonation is applied to the body part through the water in a tub, tray or tank. This method of application can be used for the treatment of hand, forearm, foot and leg. In this method ultrasound head is placed in water and moved parallel to the body part to be treated at about 1 to 2 mm away from the skin. Alternatively ultrasonic head can be just kept stationary in the water container.

Bag Method of Insonation

In bag method a plastic rubber bag filled with degassed water is placed over the body part to be treated. First couplant is smeared on the surface of bag, skin and treatment head and then the treatment head is moved over water bag. It is used for irregular surface, which can't conventionally be placed in water. Higher output may be required due to the presence of two interfaces, one between the ultrasonic head and bag and the other between bag and the body part.

Testing of Ultrasound Machine

Ultrasound machine can be tested prior to its use for the treatment purpose so as to ensure that it is working properly and emitting the ultrasonic waves. It can be tested by various ways.

Water Drops Method

Here few drops of water are splashed on the surface of the treatment head and then the output is increased momentarily. It will cause the vibration of water, which appears as if it is boiling.

Container Method

Apply the ultrasonic gel on the bottom of a suitable container and fill it with water. Place the treatment head over the bottom of the container. It produces ripples like appearance in the water when output is increased.

Thenar Eminence

Apply ultrasonic gel to your left thenar eminence. Keep the ultrasound head over this, increase the output and move the ultrasound head slowly in a circular fashion after adjusting the output by right hand. You may feel slight warmth, which suggest that the ultrasound is working properly.

Dosages of Ultrasound

In acute conditions the dose should be 0.25 to 0.5 watts/cm^2 for 2 to 3 minutes. In chronic conditions it can be increased to 0.8 to 2 watts/cm^2. Use 3 MHz for superficial lesions and 1 MHz for deep lesions. I am not aware of any strict guidelines about the number of treatments, which should be given. But usually up to 12 treatments on everyday or alternate days can be given and after 12 treatments insonation should be stopped for at least a weak before once again repeating. Alternatively you can watch the patient's symptoms and if patient complaints of deep bone pain then it suggest that there is overdose. In case of overdose occasionally the patient may have general symptoms such as fever. Following overdose, you can reduce the intensity of application on subsequent treatments, reduce the treatment time or stop the treatment with ultrasound.

PULSED ULTRASOUND

During the early use of this modality only continuous ultrasound was used and the intensity was selected in such a way that it produced the appreciable thermal change. But slowly it was recognized that non-thermal effects can have more mechanical effects and direct effects on the nerves and hence the use of lower intensity and the pulsed form came into practice. In the pulsed form of therapeutic ultrasound the output of ultrasound commences and ceases at regular interval. The pulse duration and the interval can be adjusted by pulse ratio. Pulse ratio is the ratio of pulse length duration of each pulse to the interval duration in successive pulses. Various pulse ratios commonly used are 1:1, 1:4, 1:7 and 1:10. Usually the pulse duration is 2 millisecond but the pulse interval can be varied in the multiples of 2 millisecond so as to get different ratios. When the pulse ratio is 1:1 then the output of each pulse is 2 millisecond and the interval between the pulses is also 2 millisecond, when the pulse ratio is 1: 4 that means output is 2 millisecond but the pulse interval is 8 millisecond. Pulse ratio is often termed as space ratio. Alternatively the space ratio can also be expressed in terms of duty cycle, which is the ratio of the pulse length to the total length of the pulse plus pulse interval. Thus when we choose the pulse ratio of 1:4 that means 2 millisecond pulse duration and 8 millisecond pulse interval then it means the duty cycle will be 20%. Pulsed ultrasound produces very minimal thermal effects but it produces maximal mechanical or non-thermal effects. Hence, pulsed output of the ultrasound is preferred in acute conditions, bony prominences, for phonophoresis, for mechanical effects as in case of scars and adhesions, and in an area of the treatment where the satisfactory movement of transducer is not possible as in case of coccydynia. (memory trick for you is SP, BAM where S satisfactory movement of head impossible, P for phonophoresis, B for bone, A for acute and M for mechanical effects).

Phonophoresis

It is the transfer of drugs in ointment or gel form through the skin under the influence of ultrasound. It is also called as ultrasonophoresis or sonophoresis. The initial reports about this technique appeared in 1960's and 70's. Phonophoresis is believed to be an effective method of transferring the medication into an area without having to undergo painful and sometimes poorly placed injections. By this technique the hazard of injection and accompanying apprehension can be avoided. Phonophoresis with hydrocortisone can be used in psoriasis, scleroderma, puritis and chronic tendonitis. Phonophoresis with iodine is recommended in scars, adhesive joint disorders, calcific deposits, etc. Phonophoresis with lidocaine can be used for local anesthetic effect. Phonophoresis with salicylate ointment can be used for pain relief in various musculoskeletal conditions. Personally I use piroxicam ointment for pain relief, which gives satisfactory results. For phonophoresis use lower frequencies such as 1MHz, pulsed output, higher concentration of the drug and easily soluble drugs so that desired effect can be achieved.

Combination Therapy

In order to achieve treatment goals therapeutic ultrasound can be applied in combination with other modality and this technique of applying two modalities together is termed as combination therapy. Ultrasound can be combined with surged faradic current, TENS, interferential current and iontophoresis. The concept of ultrasound and iontophoresis has got lot of practical limitations. Ultrasound with surged faradic current or single channel TENS or bipolar interferential current can be applied by placing one electrode over the convenient area and connecting the other electrode to the ultrasound applicator by means of an alligator pin or through the machine if such facility is available in the ultrasonic machine. Bearing in mind the different treatment durations of ultrasound and TENS, interferential current and faradic stimulation this technique may not be very effective.

SUMMARY

Ultrasound can produce thermal or non-thermal effects. Acoustic streaming increases the permeability of the cells. Ultrasonic therapy can be used for pain relief. Therapeutic ultrasound accelerates the healing and can be used in vast conditions. Various precautions to be taken while treating a patient with ultrasound are; check the thermal sensation prior to the ultrasound application, use the suggested levels of ultrasound dosages, move the ultrasound head, avoid superficial bony prominences, avoid excess sensation of heat during the treatment, don't keep the ultrasound head in air when the output is on, maintain the perfect contact in between the ultrasound head and the body tissues, etc. Pulsed ultrasound produces very minimal thermal effects but it produces maximal mechanical or non-thermal effects.

chapter seven

Cryotherapy

Therapeutic use of local cold application for the treatment of various diseases and disorders is known as cryotherapy. In past it was often termed as hypothermy. Personally I prefer to call it as hypothermy! Heat abstraction or cooling by cryotherapeutic agents mostly occurs by conduction except in case of vapocoolant spray. The magnitude of cooling depends on; area of body surface exposed to cold, time of exposure, temperature difference between body tissues and cooling agent, thermal conductivity of the tissues and type of cooling agent. The physics of cooling is based on Newton's law of cooling.

PHYSIOLOGICAL EFFECTS

Physiological effects of cryotherapy are reduced body temperature, reduction in blood supply, reduction in metabolism and behavioral changes.

Body Temperature

Cold causes fall in local body temperature. However, severe local cooling may result in hypothermia. Hypothermia is a condition where the core temperature is below 35°C. It may be a life-threatening situation.

Circulatory Effect

Cold application causes reflex vasoconstriction of cutaneous vessels. Application of cold causes increase in sympathetic nerves activity, smooth muscle contraction and may increase viscosity of blood. All these changes result in reduced blood flow in the area that is directly cooled. However, when the temperature is reduced below 10°C then cold induced reflex vasodilatation may occur. Reflex vasodilatation tends to occur in a cyclical manner and is believed to result from an axon reflex. Reflex vasodilatation following cold application was first recognized and reported by Lewis in 1930. The repeated cyclical vasodilatation and vasoconstriction is known as Huntington's reaction. Cooling more than 10°C causes pain. Pain impulse or afferent impulse is carried antidromically towards skin arterioles. It leads to liberation of H substance and there by vasodilatation. Once again continued cooling causes vasoconstriction and these events are repeated.

Metabolism

Cooling of tissue decreases the metabolic activity and hence the energy and oxygen requirements of cells get reduced. This effect is one of the most important effects of cryotherapy especially from the acute injury point of view.

Behavioral Changes

Person receiving cold application for prolonged time may adopt a contracted posture. Arms and legs may be drawn up to the body by which the surface area exposed to cooling can be minimized. It is said that contracted posture can reduce the heat loss by up to 60%.

THERAPEUTIC EFFECTS

Pain Relief

Cold is one of the highly effective physiotherapeutic modality in relieving pain. It is commonly used for the relief of acute pain. It can also be used for the relief of acute exacerbation of pain on the chronic background. Pain relief may occur due to counter irritation, reduced nerve conduction, decreased inflammatory process and relief of muscle spasm.

Muscle Spasm

Cryotherapy is effective in relieving the muscle spasm. Relief of spasm may occur due to decreased muscle spindle activity and secondary to the relief of pain.

Inflammation

It may bring about early resolution of inflammation by reducing vascular or cellular component of inflammation as a result of vasoconstriction.

Swelling

Cold application can reduce the swelling following an acute injury. It may be due to vasoconstriction of arterioles and reduction in extravasations of fluid into interstitial space.

Connective Tissue Extensibility

Cryotherapy increases tissue viscosity and consequently decreases the extensibility of the connective tissue. Patient may report an increase in stiffness after cold application and hence thermotherapy is a better choice in the treatment of tightness, contracture and stiffness.

Trauma

Cryotherapy is one of the very effective modality in the treatment of acute injuries. Cryotherapy reduces pain, bleeding and swelling. In addition to this, cryotherapy increases the survival rate of the tissues. Death of cells following injury may occur due to hypoxia and increased enzyme activity. Hypoxia may occur due to physical tears of blood vessels, oedema and vascular congestion. Since, the cryotherapy application reduces the metabolism and enzyme activity, the survival rate of the damaged tissues increases.

Muscle Tone

Cryotherapy can reduce the muscle tone. Hence, it is used in the treatment of spasticity. Reduction in spasticity may occur due to decreased activity of efferent gamma fibers.

Muscle Strength and Endurance

Muscle strength may increase with short-term application of cryotherapy. But on long-term application muscle strength gets reduced. However, one hour after the cessation of cooling, muscle strength may increase. Motor endurance decreases after cooling below 27°C.

Agility

Agility or motor skill reduces by cold application. Thus even though cold reduces spasticity but to teach a motor task after cold application is somewhat difficult!

Peripheral Nerves

Cold can reduce the velocity of sensory conductivity, motor nerve conductivity and synaptic activity if the temperature of the nerve decreases. Cooling below 12°C may cause paralysis of local sensory and motor nerves.

Indications

Cryotherapy is commonly used in the treatment of acute musculoskeletal injuries (0 to 72 hours), to reduce the acute pain, to reduce muscle spasticity, for relief of muscle spasm, to initiate muscle contraction, arthritis (acute onset and acute exacerbation on chronic back ground), quadriceps lag, oedema, swelling, ankle sprain, tennis elbow, Bell's palsy, post surgical pain, bed sores, etc.

Contraindication and Precautions

Cryotherapy is contraindicated in Raynaud's disease, Raynaud's phenomenon, Burger's disease, cryoglobulinaemia, paroxysmal cold haemoglobinumia, open wound (after 48 hours), regenerating peripheral nerves, vasospastic disease, impaired sensation, cold urticaria and arteriosclerosis. Precautions should be taken while treating a patient with hypertension and local cryotherapy application into an area where nerves are superficial such as medial epicondyle, axilla and head of fibula. Precautions should also be taken while treating a patient with cardiovascular disease. While treating a patient with hypertension, monitor the blood pressure through out the treatment.

Methods of Application

Vapocoolant spray, ice cube massage, cold packs, ice packs, ice towels, cold immersion, compressive cryotherapy and chemical cold packs can be used to apply cryotherapy.

Vapocoolant Sprays

Vapocoolant sprays are commonly used in the management of sports injuries. The most common type of vapocoolant spray used in physiotherapy is fluromathane. In past, ethyl chloride vapocoolant sprays were used. But ethyl chloride is flammable, explosive and should not be inhaled. Hence nowadays, ethyl chloride sprays are rarely used. The spray removes the heat from the skin underlying tissue and feels like a cool jet stream of fluid on the skin. Spray can be applied along with stretch. The advantage of the spray is, it can be used at home and it takes very little time to apply the spray.

Technique of Application

First demonstrate it to the patient by applying it on yourself. Then you can apply it on the patient by tilting the spray bottle upside down and aligning it at 30 °C to the body part, hold it at

45 cms away from the body part and then apply the spray in a parallel sweeps fashion with a speed of 10 cm per second. You can apply the spray so as to cover the area twice or thrice. This will cause adequate cooling of the body part. If more spray is indicated then the body part must be re-warmed to avoid injury to the skin.

Ice Massage

Ice massage is usually done over a small area. Ice massage is used for pain relief in local area and facilitation of muscle contraction. Muscle contraction can be facilitated by rapid and brief application over the skin dermatome. Massage with ice is simple and inexpensive. Ice cubes are easily available and hence it is one of the easily accessible modality to therapist as well as patient. It is usually applied over a bursa, tendon, muscle belly, trigger point (before deep massage) and small areas of muscle spasm. Ice massage can be taught to patients so that it can be used at home.

Technique of Application

Water can be frozen in paper cups to make handling of the ice by the physiotherapist easier. The cup is peeled back as the ice melts. As an alternative, water may be frozen in a wax or styrofoam cup with a wooden tongue stick (ice lollipops) in the middle so that the person applying ice will not get cold. Ice cubes from household freeze also can be used for ice massage. During application, a towel can be used to wipe the water seepage from the treated area because excess water will be cold and make the patient uncomfortable. The ice is rubbed over the skin by using small overlapping circles. An area of 10 to 15 cm can be treated in 5 to 10 minutes. If a larger area is involved then any other method of applying cryotherapy should be considered. The treatment takes usually 5 to 10 minutes for the area to have reduced sensation. Patient will usually experience four distinct sensations, including intense cold, numbness, burning, aching and then analgesia. When the patient touches the area and finds inability to feel the touch sensation, the treatment is completed. Ice massage produces analgesia and continues to do so for 3 to 5 minutes after treatment. To take maximum advantage of analgesic effect, manual therapy should be done immediately after the ice massage.

Cold Packs

Cold packs are canvas bags containing silicate gel. Cold packs are available in various sizes and shapes to contour the area to be treated. These packs can be stored in a special refrigeration unit or in a household freezer. Storage temperature should be –5 °C for at least two hours before use. These packs are reusable, do not reduce the skin temperature as quickly as ice bags, the patients who do not like the cold therapy can tolerate them, cold packs can easily mold to the body part and they do not open easily as ice packs.

Technique of Application

After removal of a cold pack from refrigerator, it is applied on top of the body part to be treated. Then check in between the use. For hygienic reasons, a layer of towel can be placed between the pack and the skin surface. Patient should not lie on the top of the cold pack. Many physiotherapists apply a wet towel first to the skin and then apply the cold pack and cover it with other towel or sheet to insulate the area. If the towel is wet with the room temperature or lukewarm water, the initial contact will be more comfortable for the patient. A strap can secure the cold pack so that the area is well supported. Cold packs are usually applied for 20 minutes. After the removal of cold pack from the treatment area, they should be refrozen for at least two hours before the next use of them. For the longer use, the pack should be replaced with another cold pack.

Ice Packs

Here a plastic bag is filled with crushed ice. It can be placed directly on the body part or with wet towel in between patient's skin and ice bag. Ice pack or bag treatment time ranges from 10 to 20 minutes. They are particularly of help in the treatment of patients who had undergone surgery. Ice packs in these patients can reduce the swelling and decrease pain.

Ice Towels

Superficial cooling may be achieved by the use of ice towels. Here terry towel is placed in a bucket containing flaked ice and water then wrung out and applied to the part. It may be used for 5 to 10 minutes for analgesia to occur. Larger area may be covered but the towel will need to be replaced frequently as it warms up rapidly. Treatment with ice towels can be given for up to 20 minutes. Many physiotherapists use this method for cryokinetics or cryostretching techniques.

Cold Immersion

Here extremity is immersed for 3 to 5 seconds in slush bath and then it is removed from bath. Ice immersion can be effectively used for the treatment of extremities.

Compressive Cryotherapy

Here the compressive pumps provide external pressure and cooled water to an extremity through the sleeve. It is used to reduce swelling in an area and to prevent loss of function. These machines apply intermittent pressure to the body part so as to increase the interstitial pressure and pump the fluid back into the venous system. Pressure values used to treat upper extremity are 40 to 60 mm Hg and for lower extremity approximately 60 to 80 mm Hg (10 mm less than diastolic blood pressure of the patient). Usually the on and off time ratio is 3:1. Treatment time varies and usually lasts for 10 to 15 minutes. With some larger units, two limbs may be treated simultaneously. These machines are used at sports medicine centers for the treatment of sprains, strains contusions and for reducing oedema in acute injuries. Patients with circulatory problems possibly will have extreme difficulty in tolerating this treatment.

Chemical Cold Packs

These are prepacked chemical packs that become cool when chemicals inside it are squeezed. For example, a pack with two components, one filled with water and other with ammonium nitrate which when squeezed mixes with other contents to produce cooling. These packs are expensive, can be used only once and they can be preferred when ice is not available. These packs may cause a chemical skin burn if they open accidentally. Chemical cold packs tend to cause poor cooling. These packs are too small and they are mostly used for immediate management of musculoskeletal injuries.

SUMMARY

Therapeutic use of local cold application for the treatment of various diseases and disorders is known as cryotherapy. Cold causes fall in local body temperature. Cold application can reduce the pain, muscle spasm and swelling following an acute injury. Vapocoolant spray, ice cube massage, cold packs, ice packs, ice towels, cold immersion, compressive cryotherapy and chemical cold packs can be used to apply cryotherapy. While treating a patient with hypertension, monitor the blood pressure through out the treatment.

chapter eight

Phototherapy

In this chapter, I have tried to briefly describe the photo-therapeutic modalities such as Laser, infra-red rays and ultraviolet rays. Since the use of ultraviolet rays is getting declined because of the popularity of Laser, I have briefly mentioned the production of ultraviolet rays. More details about the same can be referred from any other relevant book.

Therapeutic Laser

Laser is an acronym for light amplification by the stimulated emission of radiation. In very simple words the Laser is a beam of radiation, which is used for various purposes. Lasers are termed as magic rays since they have enormous applications in different fields. For physiotherapeutic purpose therapeutic Laser is used. Therapeutic Laser is also known as low intensity Laser, soft Laser, cold Laser, and class 3A and 3B Laser.

Historical Aspects

Historically Einstein was the first person who gave an account of stimulated emission. In 1953 Maser (Microwave amplification by stimulated emission of radiation) was discovered. In 1955 Dr. Theodore Maiman devised a working model for the production of Laser from Ruby crystal. In 1960 Bennet, Javan and Herriott discovered Helium neon Laser. In 1962 White and Ridgen produced visible red Laser with the 632.8 nm wavelength. In 1964 Block and Zueng for the first time used

Laser for surgery. From 1980's onwards, therapeutic Laser is used for physiotherapeutic applications.

Characteristics of Laser

Laser has unique characteristics, which differentiate it from other forms of light. Various characteristic features of Laser are monochromaticity, coherence and collimation. (You can remember them with CMC where C stands for coherence, M for monochromaticity and C for collimation).

Monochromaticity

Here the word mono means single and chromaticity means colour. On its emission Laser produces single pure colour. It produces single pure colour because it has one specific wavelength. Laser light entering a prism would be identical on exit because it is monochromatic. On the other hand the white light is made-up of many different colours or wavelengths and when it passes through a prism it produces a rainbow of colours.

Coherence

Laser rays are synchronous to each other. This property of synchronicity is termed as coherence. Crest and trough of individual rays matches each other. Laser rays are synchronous to each other in space, i.e. they travel in the same direction and this coherence is known as spatial coherence. Laser rays are also coherent to each other in relation to time and this type of coherence is known as temporal coherence. Analogy about the coherence can be done with army soldiers when they are marching in step in the same direction and wearing the same dress.

Collimation

Collimation is also termed as non-divergence. Laser rays travel parallel to each other rather than diverging from each other, this property is known as collimation. Collimation does not occur in other forms of light for example bulb and battery. In case of bulb and battery, the rays divert since they consists of many different wavelengths and they spread out in all directions. It is said that the Laser rays can travel up to the moon from earth in parallel to each other, with very negligible divergence.

Classification

Lasers can be roughly classified into two types such as cold Laser and hot Laser. Cold Laser is also known as low intensity Laser or therapeutic Laser. The average power of cold Laser is less than 60mw.This power is below the power, which causes tissue heating. Hot Laser is also known as high intensity Laser or surgical Laser. Here the average power is above the power, which causes tissue heating. The power of hot Laser is more than 60mw.

Types of Laser

Various types of Lasers are Helium neon Laser, Ruby Laser, Gallium Laser, Aluminum Laser, Carbon Laser and Diode Laser. Out of these helium neon Laser, which has got wavelength of 632.8 nm, is commonly used in physiotherapy.

PRODUCTION OF LASER

Principle of Production

Laser is produced from the substances, which are capable of producing Laser rays on the basis of stimulated emission of radiation.

Functional Parts

A laser device consists of three chief components such as lasing medium, energy source and mechanical structure. (Remember with MEL and not MEL GIBSON)!

Lasing medium   It is a material, which is capable of producing Laser. It may be gaseous, liquid, solid crystal or semiconductor.

Energy source   An energy source is used to excite the lasing medium. This excitation is usually electrical. It is also known as flashgun.

Mechanical structure   It is central chamber like structure, which contains the lasing medium. It has two mirrors at either end. Out of these two mirrors, one is for reflection of photons of light back and across the chamber. Other mirror in addition to reflection, serve as an exit for the out put of photons of light or Laser (Fig. 8.1).

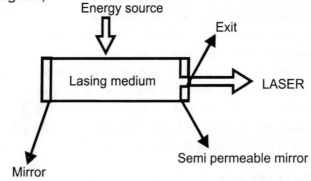

Fig. 8.1: Functional parts of therapeutic Laser device

Working

When an energy particle or the photon is applied to the atom of lasing medium it may be absorbed or reflected back. When the atom absorbs it then there is change in its electron configuration. An electron may jump from low energy level to high energy level. An atom with change in its electronic configuration is termed as an excited atom. Atom cannot remain in an excited status for long time and tries to seek its original or ground status. In order to achieve its ground status atom emits back the absorbed energy. It is emitted spontaneously and termed as spontaneous emission. If spontaneous emission is allowed to take place then Laser rays will not be emitted because the energy level necessary to achieve this may not be obtained. Hence, when the atom is in its excited state then an additional energy is applied so that the atom emits its excess of the energy immediately. This emission is known as stimulated emission. Since the emitted energy is more than what is supplied it is known as amplification. Excess of energy is emitted in form of photons of light. When these photons are emitted they are likely to be collected inside the mechanical chamber and when they move from one place to another they may hit one of the mirror. When they hit the mirror they are reflected back. Once they are reflected back they travel further through the lasing medium and increases the amplification process further. As a result more and more photons are accumulated in the mechanical chamber. When the number of photons is more than what can be accommodated in the mechanical chamber then they are emitted out of the semi permeable mirror or the mirror that has exit. The emitted photons are in form of Laser. They are carried by fiber optic cable to the probe for treatment purpose.

Effects of Laser

Pain relief: Laser has got an analgesic effect It can be used in the treatment of acute as well as chronic musculoskeletal pain. Exactly how it brings pain relief is not known. It may be as a result of endorphin secretion or due to reduced serotonin level or as per the gate control theory. Laser can be applied at trigger point, acupuncture points or at the site of pain. Personally, I never came across any patient who immediately felt the pain relief with Laser but my patients always told me that they felt pain relief after few hours. It may suggest that unlike few other electrotherapy modalities, therapeutic Laser takes some time to exhibit this effect. However, it may be confirmed in future through the research. Usually 8 to 12 treatment sessions may be required for the satisfactory pain relief but if there is no satisfactory pain relief then the Laser treatment can be stopped and any other alternative may be thought for pain relief.

Tissue Healing

It is said that Laser accelerates wounds and ulcers healing. It may be due to increased phagocytosis, facilitation of collagen synthesis, increased wound closure and wound contracture following irradiation with Laser. Cummings (1985) performed experiments on rats; he treated the artificial wounds in rats with daily Laser, alternate Laser and sham Laser. He found that there was greater healing in those rats that were treated with alternate day Laser application than daily or sham Laser. Cummings experiment may suggest that therapeutic Laser can accelerate the wounds and ulcer healing. There are various explanations or theories to explain the therapeutic Laser's efficiency in the treatment of wounds and ulcers healing.

Biostimulation theory: Laser stimulates all kinds of biological functions including biochemical, physiological and proliferative activities. It assists in proliferation of fibroblasts, re-epithelistion and remodeling. Laser also stimulates intraceflular components such as mitochondria, DNA, RNA and other substances, which are vital for the growth and repair.

Photochemical theory: Chromophores are enzymes or membrane molecules. They are photo acceptors i.e. they absorb different lights like Laser. When the Laser is absorbed by chromophores they get excited and exert biostimulative effects as above.

Indications

In physiotherapy the Laser is used mainly for pain relief and for the acceleration of the wound healing. Therapeutic Laser is used in enormous musculoskeletal conditions for pain relief. Various conditions in which Laser can be used for this purpose are rheumatoid arthritis, osteoarthritis, bursiris, pertarthritis, bicipital tendonitis, tenosynovitis, ankle sprain, trigger finger, carpal tunnel syndrome, tennis elbow, chronic low back pain, sports injuries, etc. For the healing purpose it can be used in wounds, chronic ulcers, incisions, etc.

Contraindications

Therapeutic laser is contraindicated in pregnancy especially its application around pelvis. It should not be applied at the site of tumors. Exposure to eyes with therapeutic Laser is contraindicated as it may lead to opacity of lens. It should not be applied in an area of haemorrhage, cardiac pace maker, thrombosis and unclosed fontanels of children, etc. (Memorize them with PHEN, CTC where P stands for pregnancy; H for haemorrhage, E for eyes, N for neoplasm or tumor, C for cardiac pacemaker, T for thrombosis and C for children).

Dosages and Frequency

Therapeutic Laser can be applied for 2 to 30 seconds. Few manufacturers even suggest the application of Laser up to 10 to 12 minutes! So it will be wise to calculate the dosages or follow the guidelines of the manufacturer in this aspect to get satisfactory results. Alternatively one can apply a dose of 1 to 12 J/cm^2 by using the formula.

$$\text{Energy density} = \frac{\text{Power (watts) x time (sec)}}{\text{Area (cm}^2)}$$

Therapeutic Laser in pulsed or continuous mode can be applied everyday or on alternate days for three to ten weeks.

Sites of Application

Therapeutic Laser can be applied with the point probe or cluster probe. Various sites of application for pain relief are site of pain, trigger point, tender spots, acupuncture points, etc. It can be applied by contact or non-contact technique. In contact technique Laser is applied by keeping the probe in contact with the skin or at a distance of few millimeter from the skin. (You can memorize these sites with SATT where S stands for site of pain, A for acupuncture point, T for trigger point and T for tender spots).

INFRA-RED RAYS

Infra-red rays are electromagnetic waves with wavelength of 750 to 4,00000 nm. Infra-red rays are also called as thermiogenic rays since these rays produce heat when they are absorbed by the body tissue.

Classification

Depending on wavelength, infra- red rays are classified as short wave infra-red and long wave infra-red. Short wave infra-red rays are also called as near infra-red rays. Wavelength of short wave infra-red rays ranges in between 750 to 1500 nm. Long wave infra-red rays are also called as far infra-red rays. Wavelength of these rays is above 1500 nm. Infra- red rays are also classified as, infra-red A, B and C. Infra-red A have wavelength between 750 to 1400 nm, wavelength of infra-red B is in the range of 1400 to 3000 nm and wavelength of infra- red C ranges between 3000 nm to 1 mm.

Production

Any body with high temperature than the surrounding can emit infra-red rays and hence sun is mainly the natural source of infra-red radiation. However, in physiotherapy practice various types of artificial infra- red generators are used. These generators can be divided into two types of generators; as non-luminous and luminous.

Non-luminous Generator

Non-luminous generators are also called as low temperature generators. These generators produce only infra- red rays and hence they are not visible. These generators are heated by the passage of electric current through a bare wire or carbon, held in a suitable non-conducting material like porcelain, mounted in the center of a parabolic reflector. Small non-luminous units draw 50 to 300 watts of power and larger ones draw up to 1500 watts. These generators emit only infra-red rays. All non-luminous generators emit infra-red rays in between 750 to 1500 nm. The maximum emission of the rays is around 4000 nm.

Luminous Generator

Luminous generators are also called as high temperature generators. Luminous generators emit visible rays, ultraviolet rays and infra-red rays and hence they are visible. These generators are in form of incandescent bulbs. An incandescent bulb consists of a wire filament enclosed in a glass bulb, which may or may not contain an inert gas at a low pressure. The filament is a coil of fine wires usually made of tungsten. This material tolerates repeated heating and cooling. The exclusion of air prevents the oxidation of filament, which would cause an opaque deposit to form inside the bulb. The wattage of the bulb may vary from 60 to 1000 watts, although the use of bulbs with higher wattage is discouraged because of the danger of the explosion during the treatment. Incandescent bulb is generally mounted at the center of the parabolic reflector and the reflector is mounted on an adjustable stand. All luminous generators emit the electromagnetic waves with the wavelength in between 350 to 4000 nm but the maximum emission of the rays is around 1000 nm. Accessories such as localizers, filters to filter out ultra violet rays and visible rays were used commonly in the past. However, nowaday only one accessory in form of variable resistance may be used so as to control the intensity of infra-red rays (Fig. 8.2).

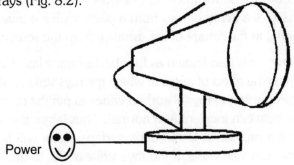

Power

Fig. 8.2: Luminous generator

Depth of Penetration

Maximum effective penetration of infra-red rays is 3 centimeter, however it may vary from 0.1 millimeter to few centimeter. It is said that infra- red rays from non-luminous generators have less depth of penetration as compared to that of luminous generators.

Laws Regulating the Absorption of Radiations

Various laws regulating the absorption of radiations including infra-red rays are Grothus law, law of inverse square, cosine law, Beer-Lambert law, Kirchhoff's law, Wien's law, Stefan Boltzman law and Arndt-Schulz principle.

Grothus law: It is also known as Grothus-Drapper law. It states that the rays must be absorbed to produce the effect and the effect will produce at that point at which the rays are absorbed. I always explain this law to my students with very simple analogy. I say you will pass the exam provided you will study and you will pass those subjects which you will study. In another words to pass you should study but by studying the electrotherapy you will pass in electrotherapy and not in any other subject. Although its not a perfect analogy, but it helps me to explain the law to my students.

Law of inverse square   Law of inverse square explains the effect of distance on the intensity of infra-red rays. It states that the intensity of a beam of rays from a point source is inversely proportional to the square of the distance from the source.

Cosine law   It is also known as Lambert's cosine law. Cosine law explains the effect of angle at which the rays strike. It states that the proportion of rays absorbed varies as per the cosine of the angle between incident and normal. Thus larger the angle at which the rays strike to the body surface, lesser will be the absorption and vice versa. If the rays strike at 90° to the body part then angle between the incident and normal or perpendicular will be zero and the cosine of 0° is maximum that is 1. Thus there will be maximum absorption if the rays will strike the body part at 90° as per this law. Hence, we always try to apply the infra-red rays in such a way that they strike at the 90° angles to the body part to be treated.

Beer-Lambert law   Degree of absorption depends on the wavelengths of radiation and nature of absorbing materials.

Kirchhoff's law   It states that good radiators are good absorbers.

Wien's law   This law states that the wavelength of maximal emission is inversely proportional to the absolute temperature of the source so that hotter the source shorter is the wavelength of emitted rays.

Stefan-Boltzman law   Stefan Boltzman law states that the output of the infra-red lamp will depend on the temperature of the element and its radiating area.

Arndt-Schulz principle   This principle states three things. Addition of a sub threshold quantity of energy wifl not cause a demonstrable change; addition of threshold and above quantity of energy will stimulate the absorbing tissue to normal function and if too great a quantity of energy is absorbed then added energy will prevent normal function or destroy tissue.

Physiological Effects

When infra- red rays are applied to the body, they are absorbed by it. As a result of absorption of infra-red rays the electromagnetic energy is converted into the thermal energy and thus heat is produced. The principle physiological effect of the infra- red rays on the body is the heat production. Other physiological effects occur as a result of heat production. Various physiological effects of infra- red rays are local rise in temperature, increased activity of sweat glands, increased metabolism, vasodilatation, relaxation of muscle tissue. On extensive or the general treatment of entire body there is general rise in body temperature and fall in blood pressure.

Therapeutic Effects

Different therapeutic effects of infra- red rays are relief of pain, muscle relaxation and increased blood supply. The analgesic effect of infra- red rays is not well understood. Mild heating with infra- red rays may cause pain relief due to sedation. But the strong heating may cause irritation and relieve the pain by counter irritation. Pain relief may occur due to relaxation of muscle spasm. Infra- red rays can relive the muscle spasm due to decreased firing of gamma spindles within the muscle. Pain relief may also occur due to removal of pain substance as a result of increased blood supply and vasodilatation if pain is associated with the accumulation of waste products.

Uses

Infra- red rays are commonly used in the treatment of subacute and chronic inflammatory conditions in areas, which are accessible to exposure. Various forms of arthritis such as osteoarthritis and rheumatoid arthritis where joints are painful and the pressure by other modality like hot packs, etc on it must be avoided then infra- red rays can be a treatment of choice.

Skin conditions such as furunculitis, folliculitis, etc can be treated with infra- red rays. Infra- red rays can be used as a preliminary modality before stretching exercises. It can also be used in the treatment of Bell's palsy for the relief of pain at the root of ear. Infra- red rays application in Bell's palsy may also be of a value since it may produce perspiration which will reduce the skin resistance and facilitate the electrical stimulation of facial muscles. Muscle spasm of traumatic and nontraumatic orthopedic origin also can be very well treated with infra-red rays.

Contraindications

Various contraindications to local heating are fever, pelvic region in pregnancy, over malignant area, impaired sensations, anesthetic area, advanced cardiac disease, eczema, dermatitis, impaired circulation, noninflammatory oedema, altered consciousness, haemorrhagic conditions, varicose veins, patients who are in extremes of age and following X-ray therapy.

Dosages on Infra-Red Rays

For acute cases irradiation with infra- red rays can be given for 10 to 15 minutes daily for 1 to 3 times as per the requirement. For chronic cases up to 30 minutes once on daily or on alternate days can be given. The infra- red generator is arranged in such a position so that it is opposite to the center of the area to be treated and the rays strike at right angles. Irradiation can be applied at a distance of 50 to 75 cm. During irradiation of the face cover the face, eyes and hair. Eyes should be protected by moist cotton packs otherwise opacities of lens may occur.

Hazards of Infra-Red Irradiation

Although not very common but few hazards or dangers due to infra- red irradiation may occur. They are burns, electric shock, edema, overdose, faintness, headache, injury to eyes permanent pigmentation, blisters, etc. These dangers can be prevented by number of precautions such as regularly checking the infra- red generator for electrical safety.

ULTRAVIOLET RAYS

Ultraviolet rays are invisible rays with wavelengths between 10 to 400 nm.Ultraviolet rays are of three types such as ultraviolet A, B and C. Although ultraviolet rays are emitted by sun, but for physiotherapeutic treatment purpose ultraviolet generators produce them. Most of these generators produce ultraviolet rays from mercury. Various generators such as high pressure mercury vapor lamp, low pressure mercury vapor lamp, fluorescent tubes, Kromayer lamp, PUVA box, theraktin tunnel, etc. can be used for physiotherapeutic applications.

Physiological Effects of Ultraviolet Rays

Ultraviolet rays can produce localized and generalized physiological effects. Various physiological effects of ultraviolet rays are erythema reaction, thickening of the epidermis, desquamation, pigmentation, esophylactic effect, antibiotic effect, vitamin D formation and general tonic effect.

Erythema Reaction

Absorption of ultraviolet rays produces erythema reaction characterized by redness of the skin. This erythema is produced mainly because of ultraviolet rays with wavelengths in between 250 to 297 nm. The severity of erythema depends on the intensity of chemical reaction produced by ultraviolet rays. Intensity of reaction is higher if the duration of exposure is higher and the distance between the ultraviolet ray source and the body tissue is lesser. If the intensity of irradiation with ultraviolet rays is less then it may not produce visible red colour of the skin. Erythema occurrence is mediated through the chemical changes. These chemical changes are likely to occur due to release of H substance as a result of irradiation. Release of H substance produces triple response. Triple response is characterized by dilatatation of capillaries, dilatation of arteries and exudation. These changes are similar to inflammation and hence erythema can be termed as inflammatory reaction. Erythema reaction occurs after 12 hours of irradiation. Depending upon severity of chemical reaction and cessation time, erythema is divided into four degrees.

First degree erythema (E1)   It is characterized by slight reddening of the skin with no irritation or soreness. It subsides in 24 hours.

Second degree erythema (E2)   It is characterized by more reddening of the skin with slight irritation. It subsides in two or three days.

Third degree erythema (E3)   There is obvious reddening of the skin, which is hot, sore and edematous. The reaction lasts for about a week.

Fourth degree erythema (E4)   Here all the third degree erythema changes are present but in addition to this there is blister formation.

Thickening of the Epidermis

Ultraviolet rays causes damage to the superficial cells. It is followed by increased production of these cells, which tend to cause the thickening of the epidermis.

Desquamation

It is the casting off dead cells from the surface of the body. Ultraviolet rays causes damage to the cells, these damaged cells are casted off and the process by which the dead cells are casted off is known as peeling.

Pigmentation

Ultraviolet rays may cause conversion of the amino acid tyrosine into the pigment melanin. Extent of pigmentation varies as per the individual; it is more in those with dark skin than with fair skin.

Esophylactic Effect

It is the increased body's resistance to infection as a result of ultraviolet rays action on reticuloendothelial system. Some retiucloendothelial cells are situated in the superficial tissues. Ultraviolet rays can affect superficially situated reticuloendothelial cells and reduce the irritability threshold of these cells, so that antibodies are produced more readily in response to bacteria and their toxins.

Bactericidal Effect

Short ultraviolet rays can destroy bacteria and other microorganisms commonly found in wounds. Fourth degree erythema (E4) dose can effectively destroy all such organisms found in wounds.

Vitamin D Formation

Ultraviolet rays may cause conversion of 7 dehydrocholesterol into vitamin D. 7- DHC is present in sebum and hence this reaction may occur at the surface of the skin or in superficial layers of the skin.

General Tonic Effect

General tonic effect such as improved appetite, improved sleep and reduced irritability may occur due to ultraviolet rays irradiation. However there is no evidence for this.

THERAPEUTIC EFFECTS OF ULTRAVIOLET RAYS

Various therapeutic effects of ultraviolet rays are counterirritation, increased blood supply, destruction of bacteria, tissue destruction and desquamation.

Counterirritation

Ultraviolet irradiation may cause irritation of superficial sensory nerve endings and hence may relieve the pain through counterirritation. Usually a third degree erythema dose is required for this purpose.

Increased Blood Supply

Ultraviolet rays increase the blood supply to the skin as a result of erythema reaction. It can be used in the treatment of certain conditions such as psoriasis, acne, alopecia and chilblains.

Destruction of Bacteria

Ultraviolet rays can destroy bacteria. Hence, ultraviolet irradiation can be used in the treatment of superficial bacterial infections such as infected wounds, adenitis and acne.

Tissue Destruction

Ultraviolet rays damages and destroy the superficial cells. It may be applied to sluggish wounds for this purpose.

Desquamation

This casting off reaction of ultraviolet rays is of value in the treatment of acne.

INDICATIONS AND CONTRAINDICATIONS

Ultraviolet rays are used in the treatment of psoriasis, acne, bedsores, alopecia, chilblains, sluggish wounds, adenitis, infected wounds and marasmus. However, ultraviolet ray irradiation is contraindicated in presence of fever, acute eczema, irradiation into thoracic region in presence of pulmonary tuberculosis, following X-ray therapy, hypersensitive individuals, systemic lupus erythematosus, photoallergy and skin grafts.

HAZARDS AND PRECAUTIONS

Hazards of ultraviolet irradiation are conjunctivitis, overdose, electric shock, burns and chilling sensation. Avoiding the exposure of eyes by using dark glasses or glasses made-up of Chances Crooke A glass and using shades around the lamp with the help of clothe can prevent it. Over dose can be prevented by carrying out test dosages on patient before application. Test dosage can be carried out so as to find out time duration of irradiation at a particular distance to produce El reaction. Once we know die El reaction then one can calculate the time period required at the same distance or any other distance by calculations like E2 is 2.5 times El, E3 is 5 times El and E4 is 10 times El. The dose can also be calculated at any other distance by using the following formula;

$$\text{New dose} = \frac{\text{Old dose X New distance}^2}{\text{Old distance}^2}$$

Electric shock can be prevented by regular checkups for leakage of current and proper earthing. Burns may occur if hot part of the lamp was touched. Asking the patient not to touch any part of the ultraviolet generator can prevent electric shock. Chill may occur if total body irradiation is carried out and when the treatment room is too cold. Maintaining the adequate room temperature and simultaneous irradiation of patient with infrared rays can prevent it

PUVA AND IONOZONE THERAPY

It is a treatment technique used for the treatment of various diseases in which ultraviolet rays are applied after giving psolaren tablet or after applying psolaren ointment. It is commonly called by its acronym PUVA (psolaren and ultravioletA). PUVA therapy is used for the treatment of leucoderma, eczema, psoriasis, uriticaria pigmentosa and cutaneous T cell lymphoma. Ionozone therapy is a treatment technique characterized by the use of ultraviolet rays, ionized water and ozone obtained from the passage of steam over mercury vapor lamp. For this purpose, special apparatus called ionozone therapy machine is used. Ionozone therapy is used for relief of pain, increase in superficial blood flow, increase in metabolic processes, increase in oxidation processes and bactericidal effect. Stitch abscess, open wounds, varicose ulcers, diabetic ulcers, pressure sores and acne can be effectively treated by ionozone therapy. In the treatment of these conditions ionozone therapy can be applied for 10 to 30 minutes at 30 to 50 cm distance from the nozzle of the ionozone therapy apparatus.

SUMMARY

Laser is an acronym for light amplification by the stimulated emission of radiation. Therapeutic Laser is mainly used for pain relief and acceleration of healing. Therapeutic Laser can be applied with the point probe or cluster probe. Infra-red rays are also called as thermiogenic rays. Various laws regulating the absorption of radiations including the infra-red rays are Grothus law, law of inverse square, Cosine law, Beer-Lambert law, Kirchhoff's law, Wien's law, Stefan Boltzrnan law and Arndt-Schulz principle. Various therapeutic effects of infrared rays are relief of pain, muscle relaxation and increased blood supply. Ultraviolet rays are of three types such as ultraviolet A, B and C. Absorption of ultraviolet rays produces erythema reaction characterized by redness of the skin. Ultraviolet rays may increase vitamin D formation and exert abiotic effect.

chapter nine

Safety Precautions in Electrotherapy

INTRODUCTION

In past there were accidental reports of electrocution during diagnostic and routine treatment with machines that works on electricity. Although there is not a single reliable and official statistic report available in our country, it seems sensible that an extra caution must be taken, whenever electrical safety codes and their implementation are as not strictly enforced as it is in more advanced countries.

I would like to share one of my experiences pertaining to the leakage of the current. This patient was a pretty married woman who had wrist pain. To alleviate her wrist pain I started treating her with an electrically operated and programmed instrument, which could offer TENS. I used to put the electrodes first then switch on the mains, set the parameters and increase the intensity. But when the treatment was over this machine would reduce the intensity to zero automatically and hence I tried to lift the electrodes and then switched off the machine. To my surprise when I touched her forearm I got shock like sensation. This happened successively for three days of treatment and then I shared this information to my colleagues who kept laughing at this. I decided to check whether there was leakage of current with the tester and to my surprise the tester was glowing in both the out put terminals of this machine where electrodes were to be connected. Then we called electrician who found that there was real leakage due to heavy raining and some fault in voltage stabilizer. Then I concluded that compared to my patient I was very sensitive to the leakage of current. Nowadays, I don't really get surprised with this thing but I call the electrician immediately without fail.

Physiotherapist working in a hospital or clinical set-up frequently uses modalities, which are electrically operated. Therefore, there is a great need for physiotherapist to be aware of the potential electrical hazards to patients as well as therapist. In 1998 I presented a paper based on questionnaire research, in Indian Association of Physiotherapists conference at Thiruvanathapuram (36th IAP conference, 25th Jan 1998) on *Implication of Informed Consent in Electrotherapy.* The outcome of this study was that all the respondents (100%) felt that we should take an informed consent from patients prior to the use of electrotherapy modalities. 73.34% respondents felt that it would protect physiotherapists from malpractice as well as accidental hazards, 20% felt that it would protect physiotherapists from only accidental hazards while, 6.66% felt that it would protect physiotherapists from only malpractice! Since this study included only 30 physiotherapists and response rate was 50%, a major study in this aspect in future may give us better insight.

CAUSES AND TYPES OF HAZARDS

Various causes of electrical hazards are worn out power cords, broken plugs, faulty lamp sockets, incorrectly wired outlets, leakage of current, defect in circuit, absence of earthing, defective electrical receptacles or sockets, breakage of power cord, etc. Types of hazards due to the use of electrotherapeutic modalities ate electric shock, electrocution, thermal burns, electrochemical bums, scalds, etc. Physiological effects of shock can vary with the magnitude of the current. *With* 0.1 milliamperes the shock is imperceptible, with 1 to 15 milliamperes it produces tingling sensations and muscle contractions, with 15 to 100 milliamperes it produces painful electrical shock, with 100 to 200 milliamperes it can produce cardiac or respiratory arrest and with more than 200 milliamperes it produces instant tissue burning and destruction.

Safety Precautions

There are many more safety precautions and it may be difficult to remember them. Hence, I have divided these precautions into three areas such as equipment purchase, earthing and voltage stabilizer, maintenance and safety precautions to be taken by physiotherapist.

Equipments purchase: Do not buy the cheapest equipments since they me be the most expensive to operate. Read the instruction manual before operating. Check the unit at the time of delivery and if there is any defect then exchange the unit. Ask for performance and safety check as a condition of sale.

Earthing and Stabilizer

There should be proper earthing connected to all the electrotherapy equipments working on electricity. Ground fault interrupter circuit should be used. You should have either separate or central voltage stabilizer for your clinic or department so as to avoid voltage surge and thereby discomfort to the patient while receiving electrical stimulation, absurd performance by the equipment and damage to equipments. I have witnessed one situation where traction machine (with microprocessor circuit) pulled one of the patient's neck with maximal weight than what it was assigned to do due to voltage surge. Switches should break the live wire. Fuses should be on live wire so that if a large current passes then the fuse blows and stop the current flow.

Maintenance

Try to have a maintenance contract with the manufacturers for yearly services after the warranty period. Routine maintenance check-up should be performed on all electrical equipments. Yearly maintenance check-up by biomedical engineer should be done. Dated inspection sticker should be affixed to all electrical units.

Physiotherapist: Physiotherapist should not use the electrical equipments near objects or environment that draw the current post sign notifying usage of equipment that interfere with pacemakers and hearing aids. Inspect the skin after every treatment. Unplug units that are not in use. Familiarize yourself with problems of electrical hazards. Physiotherapist who doesn't have sufficient knowledge and experience on electrical matters should not attempt to personally repair equipment failures however minor it is. Call expert like your hospital electrician or biomedical engineer to check the equipment for breakage. Equipment with questionable performance is noted, labelled and turned off and disconnected immediately from patient. Avoid use of extension cords. Never use the cheater adopters allowing three pronged plugs to be used in two prong receptacles. Use of under grounded electrical equipments must be avoided. Disconnect the instrument form the wall socket by pulling the connector and not the cable. Avoid spilling of water or normal saline during electrical stimulation over the stimulator. Use surgical rubber gloves when handling ultrasound for under water use. Use the tester to check for leakage of current. Attend seminars and lectures dealing with electrical safety. Keep update information about new instruments. Whenever you buy new equipment then read the instruction manual or get the training before operating it frequently check the integrity of plug cords, electrical stimulation leads for fraying or disruption. Report the loose gripping connections between plug and receptacles and get it repaired. Do not permit your patient to touch the apparatus during the treatment. Take special care when you administer the treatment through bath, as there is always possibility of easy earth connections. Bath must be of an insulating material and leaking bath tray or tub or tank should not be used.

SUMMARY

Various causes of electrical hazards are worn out power cords, broken plugs, faulty lamp sockets, incorrectly wired outlets, leakage of current, defect in circuit, absence of earthing, defective electrical receptacles or sockets, breakage of power cord, etc. With 0.1 mA the shock is imperceptible, with 1 to 15 mA it produces tingling sensations and muscle contractions, with 15 to 100 mA it produces painful electrical shock, with 100 to 200 mA, it can produce cardiac or respiratory arrest and with more than 200 mA it produces instant tissue burning and destruction. There should be proper earthing connected to all the electrotherapy equipments working on electricity. Routine maintenance check-up should be performed on all electrical equipments.

chapter ten

Clinical Decision Making in Electrotherapy

INTRODUCTION

One can decide about which modality should be chosen in a particular instance but the real art lies not in selecting the modality but selecting it so that it fetch positive outcome. Several modalities are available and each one for them has ability to reduce amount of discomfort that a patient may be experiencing. There is overlapping of clinical effects and results of these modalities. The questions like what should I choose, when should I choose, how should I choose, should I follow the same sequence again and so on arises during clinical situations. Here are some personal comments that may help you in clinical decision-making. But remember that whatever you think is right for your patient and you try to follow the same. Hence it's totally upto you whether to follow my suggestions or not.

Suggestions for Clinical Decision Making

I take into consideration my previous experience of similar patient, previous experience of patient if he has taken the physiotherapy treatment, irritability of the patient, underlying pathology, contraindications, medical condition of the patient, special request by the referring clinician, patient's comfort, treatment time, area to be treated, depth of penetration, equipment availability, reliability of the equipment, familiarity with equipment, proved outcome, professional suggestions and patient's response.

Physiotherapist's Previous Experience

Most of the physiotherapists decide about the electrotherapeutic modalities on the basis of their experience with similar kind of case. If their previous patient had responded to a modality then they prefer the same one for their next patient with similar clinical problem.

Patient's previous experience   Patient's previous experience with modality also can be taken into consideration while making a clinical decision about the modality that is to be selected. If your patient had beneficial effect with a particular modality then use that modality. On the other hand if your patient had adverse effect or no response with that modality then try to avoid the use of same modality.

Irritability   If the condition is highly irritable then electro-analgesic modalities (such as TENS, interferential, etc) and cold therapy can be preferred.

Underlying pathology If underlying pathology is very acute then cryotherapy and electro analgesic-modalities can be preferred, in subacute superficial heating modalities and in chronic cases deep heating modalities can be preferred. I always tell my students to note the local temperature. I suggest them to choose cold if the area to be treated is hot (increased local temperature) because of underlying pathology and if the local temperature is not increased then choose the hot!

Contraindications Rule out the possibility of the contraindications for the modality you have decided to use. If it's contraindicated then think of any other modality that is not contraindicated for that patient. For instance you decided to use short wave diathermy but you came to know that your patient has got metal implant in the area of treatment then you can choose a modality like infrared or hot pack rather than short wave diathermy.

Medical condition of patient   Clinical decision-making should also be done on the basis of underlying medical/ surgical condition of the patient. For instance if the patient is referred to you for pain management but the underlying cause of the pain is tumor then many of the electrotherapeutic modalities are contraindicated. In this case you may think about local application of TENS rather than those modalities that are contraindicated.

Special request   Sometimes the clinical decision-making about the use of electrotherapy modality is done on the basis of special request by referring clinician.

Comfort of the patient   If a patient feels comfortable with a modality then try to use the same. Few patients doesn't like current treatment and are scared of the same then try to choose any other modality that won't cause electrical stimulation of sensory nerves and thereby discomfort to your patient.

Treatment time   If you have very less treatment time available for the treatment of your patient as in case of acute sports injuries then choose an electrotherapy modality which requires less treatment time. For instance, vapocoolant spray and laser can be preferred in sports injuries.

Area to be treated   If area to be treated is very small then focal treatment such as therapeutic ultrasound can be preferred. If it is larger then other modality like short wave diathermy can be used.

Depth of penetration   Modality selection can be done on the basis of depth of penetration. For instance if you have a patient with periostitis then choose therapeutic ultrasound which has highest depth of penetration of all the modalities.

Equipment availability   Clinical decision-making can also be done on the basis of equipment availability. For instance you wanted to use long wave diathermy but if it is not available in your clinic or hospital then you should think of any other modality that can have similar effect.

Reliability of equipment   You should choose that equipment which gives you a reliable performance.

Familiarity   You should not use equipment unless you don't get familiarized with its controls and parameters settings.

Proved outcome   If the treatment outcome is well proved and clinically established then you should try to prefer that modality. For example therapeutic ultrasound is proved better in the treatment of calcific bursitis and plantar fascitis, etc. then try to use the same in these conditions.

Professional suggestions   Always follow the professional suggestions and guidelines for the use of therapeutic modalities while treating various clinical conditions.

Patient's response   If your patient responds positively to the modality you have chosen then continue the use of it otherwise think whether you should alter the dosiometry or you should prefer other modality.

SUMMARY

Physiotherapist's previous experience of similar patient, previous experience of patient if he has taken the physiotherapy treatment, irritability of the patient, underlying pathology, contraindications, medical condition of the patient, special request by the referring clinician, patient's comfort, treatment time, area to be treated, depth of penetration, equipment availability, reliability of the equipment familiarity with equipment, proved outcome, professional suggestions and patient's response can be taken into consideration while making clinical decisions.

chapter eleven

Biofeedback

INTRODUCTION

Since 1960's biofeedback has got recognized as a clinical tool in clinical medicine, behavioral medicine, physiotherapy and rehabilitation medicine. Information regarding history of biofeedback is not readily available to physiotherapists and it appears to be not widely described. Various references suggests that the systematic study of biofeedback started in 1960's with attempts to train voluntary control of autonomic function such as heart rate and blood pressure. Although significant improvement may occur in different conditions, how far the biofeedback devices are effective should be verified by repeated researches in this field. In general, biofeedback can be defined as the process of furnishing an individual with information about body functioning so as to get some voluntary control over it. This information regarding body functioning can be given to the individual via visual or auditory signal through a suitable instrument. In order to understand the biofeedback, please refer the Figure 11.1.

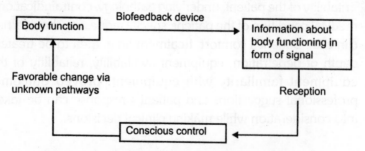

Fig. 11.1: Schematic diagram of biofeedback

Types of Biofeedback

Just a brief outline of these biofeedback devices is given here and the reader is requested to refer any comprehensive book on this subject for more details. Various forms of biofeedback devices are as follows.

Myoelectric Feedback

This is also known EMG biofeedback EMG biofeedback is commonly used in physiotherapy. A set of surface electrodes is placed on the skin over chosen muscle or muscle group to detect electrical signals associated with muscle contraction. These signals are amplified and translated into simple auditory and visual signals that are very easy to understand This auditory or visual information concerning the state of muscle tension or relaxation is provided to the patient via auditory or visual display. Auditory display is in form of clicks or buzzing sound and visual display is inform of movement of meter needle or glowing of the lights or computer display rather than oscilloscope trace. As this display bears an approximate relationship to the magnitude of the muscle contraction causing it, re-education of the muscles is possible. In other words, it is possible to get the desired response from muscle with this device by increasing or decreasing the activity of these muscles. EMG biofeedback is commonly used in the treatment of recovering peripheral nerve injuries, writer's cramp, blepharospasm, training specific muscle activity after tendon or muscle transplant and dystonic conditions. It is also used to improve shoulder control, to re-educate dorsiflexion of foot and to reduce spasticity of plantar flexors in hemiplegia. Biofeedback devices can also be used in the treatment of spasticity in cerebral palsy and multiple sclerosis.

Postural Biofeedback

Scoliosis biofeedback device is a modified orthotic device that is beneficial in the treatment of scoliosis. Whenever the scoliotic wearer leans against a thoracic pad of this device he receives the auditory signals which encourages him to straighten the spine. Inclination monitor is helpful in postural control. Inclination monitor device can be worn any where on the trunk and senses a tilt from vertical head position trainer device can be used in cerebral palsy children with delayed head control. The tremor monitor device measures the hand steadiness and is used to improve hand control.

Feedback Goniometers

These devices monitor the joint angles. Elbow angle monitor is used to increase range of motion of elbow joint. Knee angle monitor is useful in prevention of hyperextension at knee. Ankle angle monitors can be used in the treatment of foot drop during swing phase of the gait. Hip rotation monitor device measures internal and external rotation of the foot with respect to the pelvis and may be useful in correction of gait deviations such as excessive internal or external rotation of hip.

Pressure or Force Biofeedback

These devices monitors the pressure or force. The limb load monitor consists of a shoe insole with pressure sensor, which senses the amount of the weight applied to it. It is used to encourage the patients like hemiplegics to put more weight on affected leg while standing or walking. Prosthetic grip strength monitor is applied to myoelectric upper limb prosthesis for strengthening of the grip.

Orofacial Control Devices

Orofacial control devices can be used in the treatment of orofacial problems in cerebral palsy children. Jaw closure monitor is helpful in drooling problem. Wet chin alarm device detect "the build up of saliva and gives auditory signals to wearer so as to control it. Palatograph detects the position of tongue on the roof of mouth.

Toilet training devices: Toilet training biofeedback can improve the toilet activities. The enuresis alarm detects the presence of the urine and sound on alarm. It works by detecting changes in electrode conductance when moisture is present between electrodes. It is useful in the treatment of bed-wetting. Perineometer is used in re-education of pelvic floor muscles in case of incontinence. It works by measuring the pressure or electrical activity of pelvic floor muscles through vaginal or rectal pressure probes or electrodes.

Stress related devices: These biofeedback devices minimize the stress by increasing relaxation. EMG biofeedback device can be used in the treatment of tension headache. For this, relaxation of the occipitofrontalis muscle and posterior neck muscles is taught, since it is believed that the cause of this type of headache is tension in these muscles. The galvanic skin response monitor detects the changes in conductance of hand caused by the activity of sweat glands. Since the skin conductance is associated with arousal, patient can learn to reduce arousal to achieve whole body relaxation. It may be valuable in reducing spasm in cerebral palsy in addition to inducing relaxation in normal individuals. For epileptic patients a biofeedback device that detects the special rhythm in EEG can be used to reduce the frequency of epileptic fits.

Cardiovascular Biofeedback

In patients with hypertension, blood pressure can be monitored and displayed to the patient who gradually learns some voluntary control over it. Biofeedback can also be used in the treatment of cardiac arrhythmias. Here the heart rate is monitored and displayed to the patient who can learn some voluntary control over it. In Raynaud's disease the temperature of finger is monitored and patient attempts to increase the temperature voluntarily.

Treatment Duration

There are no specific criteria for the duration of the treatment with biofeedback devices. However, favorable results are likely to occur with the use of the biofeedback devices for 10 to 30 minutes per day.

Advantages and Disadvantages

Advantages

Biofeedback provides corrective information to the patient immediately. Patient gets involved actively in his own treatment Biofeedback may not require sophisticated understanding of the skill by patients. Biofeedback devices can be used during on going activities. It may save physiotherapist's time.

Disadvantages

Biofeedback treat symptoms and not the underlying cause of symptoms. Biofeedback training or treatment is uneconomical as all of these devices are not available commercially at all the places. Biofeedback devices are unacceptable to patients who won't like to put wires and electronic boxes over their body. Sometimes physiotherapists may need special training for the use of biofeedback. Biofeedback could be just a form of training rather than treatment.

SUMMARY

Biofeedback is the process of furnishing an individual with information about body functioning so as to get some voluntary control over it. This information regarding body functioning can be given to the individual via visual or auditory signal through a suitable instrument. Various forms of biofeedback include myoelectric feedback, postural biofeedback, feedback goniometers, pressure or force biofeedback, orofacial control devices, toilet training devices, stress related devices, cardiovascular biofeedback, etc. These biofeedback devices provide corrective information to the patient immediately. There are no specific criteria for the duration of the treatment with biofeedback devices. Biofeedback devices may be unacceptable to patients who won't like to put wires and electronic boxes over their body.

Appendix

LOCATION OF MOTOR POINTS

You can use these guidelines to find out the motor points during therapeutic stimulation purpose. These guidelines may work in few individuals. I suggest you to try with these guidelines just three times and if you don't get the motor point then you can search at any other location by trial and error method.

Face

Frontalis   About halfway between hairline and center of eyebrow.

Corrugator   Above the outer third of the superciliary arch.

Orbicularis oculi   Just below and lateral to outer angle of eye.

Procerus   On side of nose just below inner angle of eye.

Nasalis   Just above ala of nose.

Orbicularis oris   Upper point can be located at about halfway between angle of mouth and tip of nose and the lower point approximately in the same position below mouth.

Risodus   About one finger's breadth lateral to the angle of mouth.

Buccinator   About two fingers width lateral to the angle of mouth.

Mentalis   Midline near prominence of chin.

Forearm and Hand

Abductor pollicis brews   Over the thenar eminence about an inch from the wrist approximately at the center of the thenar prominence.

Flexor pollicis brevis   Upper border of thenar eminence.

Opponens pollicis   Thenar eminence near wrist, press the electrode in the thenar eminence since it's a deeply situated muscle.

Adductor pollicis   In the web between thumb and index finger equally accessible on dorsal or palmar aspects.

Abductor digiti minimi   About a finger breadth distal to wrist on ulnar border.

Flexor digiti minimi   To the radial side of point for opponens digiti minimi.

Opponens digiti minimi   About halfway between web of the little finger and the wrist, press the electrode since it's a deeply situated muscle.

Lumbricals   About three fingers breadth proximal to each interdigital web. There is one point for each one of four muscles.

Palmar interossei   About one finger breadth proximal to interdigital webs on palmar aspect. There is one point for each of these muscles. Very small electrode should be used

Dorsal interossei   About one or two fingers breadth proximal to finger webs on dorsal aspect. There is one point for each muscle. Press the electrode.

Pronator teres   About an inch below elbow and an inch from midline on ulnar side.

Flexor carpi radialis   About 1/3rd down from the elbow to the ulnar side of the midline.

Flexor digitorum superficfalis   Middle and lower third of forearm on ulnar side. Four points can be located on a diagonal line from medial condyle of elbow to middle of wrist.

Palmaris longus   Just inside to the point of flexor carpi ulnaris.

Flexor carpi ulnaris   About three finger's breadth below elbow on extreme ulnar border.

Flexor pollicis longus   About two inches above wrist near radial border.

Flexor digitorum profundus   About three fingers' breadth below elbow crease just to ulnar side of midline. Less accessible than superficialis.

Pronator quadratus   At about three fingers width proximal to wrist crease press the electrode about medial to midline.

Brachioradialis   At about three fingers width from elbow crease with forearm in midprone position.

Extensor carpi radialis longus   Below and to the radial side of olecranon.

Extensor carpi radialis brevis   A few inches below the point for longus.

Extensor digitorum   On a line from radial side of the elbow to the middle of the wrist; three points in the middle third of this line.

Extensor digiti minimi   Dorsal mid forearm at ulnar side.

Extensor carpi ulnaris   About three inches below olecranon and on ulnar side of midline.

Anconeus   About two inches above olecranon process.

Supinator   Difficult to find but can be tried on the dosrsum of the hand at two fingers distal to elbow crease at midline.

Abductor pollicis longus   Near radial border about halfway between elbow and wrist.

Extensor pollicis longus   About three fourths of the way down from the elbow on ulnar side. Sometimes difficult to find.

Extensor pollicis brevis   In middle at about two-thirds down from elbow.

Extensor indicis   About halfway between elbow and wrist just ulnar to midline.

Leg and Foot Muscles

Tibialis anterior   About a hand's breadth below lower angle of patella and one finger lateral to tibial crest.

Extensor digitorum longus   About one finger below prominence of fibular head and slightly towards midline.

Extensor digitorum brevis   On the dorsum of foot about two fingers below angle formed by leg and foot. There are two motor points for this muscle.

Extensor hallucis longus   About three fingers above ankle at about midline.

Gastroenemius   Medial point at about eight fingers below popliteal crease near medial border of calf. Lateral point at about five inches below popliteal crease near lateral border of calf.

Soleus   About two-thirds the way down from knee, on point about three fingers each side of midline.

Flexor hallucis longus   About three fingers behind and above lateral malleolus.

Flexor digitorum longus   In fossa behind medial malleolus, about three fingers above and medial to achillis tendon.

Tibialis posterior   About two thirds down from the knee medial to soleus against the tibia.

Peroneus longus   Just below head of fibula.

Peroneus brevis   About a hand's breadth above and lateral to external malleolus.

Abductor hallucis   Medial border of foot arch, about two fingers below medial malleolus.

Flexor digitorum brevis   Just forward to center of sole.

Flexor hallucis brevis   About three fingers from middle of base of great toe in sole.

Abductor digiti minimi   In front of heel near lateral border.

Physiotherapy for Peripheral Nerve Injuries

The outline of physiotherapy treatment following peripheral nerve injury is described here. It consists of electrical stimulation, passive movements, splints, counseling and reassurance (You can memorize with CRESP where C stands for counseling, R for reassurance, E for electrical stimulation, S for splint and P for passive movements).

Electrical stimulation Electrical stimulation is given to the paralyzed muscles so as to maintain nutrition of muscles and prevent the disuse atrophy, degeneration and fibrosis. Selection of the current can be done on the basis of faradic interrupted direct current test.

Passive movements   Passive movements should be given to the affected joints so as to maintain the range of motion and there by prevention of overstretching of paralyzed muscles, tightness and contracture of intact antagonist muscles.

Splints/orthoses   Splints or orthoses should be advised so as to preserve the function and avoid overstretching of affected muscles by antagonist.

Counseling   Counseling of the patient should be done. It may involve instructions about prevention of injury to desensitized parts.

Reassurance   Reassure that the loss of function and sensation could be temporary and will return within few weeks to few months.

Classification of Nerve Injuries

Peripheral nerve injuries mainly occur due to pressure, trauma and exposure to cold. (Memorize with CPT its not abbreviation for chest physiotherapy but here C for cold, P for pressure and T for trauma). These peripheral nerve injuries can be classified so as to get an idea about their nature of injury, severity, prognosis and treatment planning. There are various classifications of peripheral nerve injuries such as Sheddon's classification, Sunderlands classification and Spencer's classification.

Sheddon's classification   As per Sheddon's classification peripheral nerve injuries can be classified as neuropraxia, axonotmesis and neurotmesis.

Neuropraxia Is a type of peripheral nerve injury characterized by transient physiological conduction block without any significant pathological changes. For example neuropraxic lesion of the facial nerve in Bell's palsy. Neuropraxia causes transient ischemia at the point of nerve injury, which leads to degeneration of myelin sheath and hence physiological conduction block occurs at the site of nerve injury. However, there is no loss of axonal continuity, there is no Wallerian degeneration. Nerve deficit is completely reversible.

Axonotmesis   It is a type of nerve injury characterized by intrathecal rupture of axons or nerve fibers. For example the radial nerve injury associated with fracture of the shaft of humerus. Pathologically there is rupture of the nerve fibers but the myelin sheath remains intact. Axon undergoes the Wallerian degeneration in its distal cut end and upto the first node of Ranvier proximally. There is complete loss of nerve conduction distal to the injury.

Neurotmesis   It is a type of peripheral nerve injury characterized by rupture of both nerve sheath as well as nerve fiber. Neruotmesis may be partial or complete. In partial neurotmesis only the portion of nerve is cut. In complete neurotmesis nerve is divided across its whole thickness. Example of this nerve injury can be, complete ulnar nerve cut as a result of glass cut injury. Pathological changes in form of Wallerian degeneration occur in distal part of the cut end of the nerve and up to the first node of Ranvier proximally. Disruption of the Schwan cells and endoneurimal connective tissue also occurs. There is complete loss of conduction distal to the site of nerve injury.

Sunderland's classification   Peripheral nerve injuries are classified as first degree, second degree, third degree, fourth degree and fifth degree injuries. First and second degree injuries are similar to neuropraxia and axonotmesis respectively. Neurotmesis type of injuries comprise third, fourth and fifth degree injuries. In third degree injury there is interruption of nerve fibers. In fourth degree there is connective tissue damage in addition to interruption of nerve fibers. In fifth degree there is severance of nerve in addition to above changes.

Schaumburg, Spencer and Thomas classification   This classification classifies the peripheral nerve injuries in to class one, class two and class three types of injuries. Class one is same as that of neuropraxia, class two is similar to axonotmesis and class three is like neurotmesis.

Glossary

Acne An inflammatory disease of the skin with the formation of an eruption of papules or pustules.

Acute pain A short sharp cutting pain. It is usually associated with acute inflammation.

Accommodation Adaptation by the sensory receptors to various stimuli over an extended period of time.

Acupuncture Treatment of human ailments by inserting fine needles in to the acupuncture points.

Adhesion Fibrous band that holds together tissues that are normally separated.

Adenitis Inflammation of a gland.

Alternating current Current that periodically changes its polarity or direction of flow.

Alopecia Baldness, absence of hair from skin areas where it is normally present.

Amplitude The intensity of current flow as indicated by. the height of the waveforms from baseline.

Analgesia Absence of pain or loss of sensibility of pain.

Anesthesia Partial or complete loss of sensations with or without loss of consciousness as a result of disease, injury or administration of an anesthetic agent usually by an injection or inhalation.

Anode   Positively charged electrode.

Bursitis   Inflammation of a bursa especially located between bony prominences and muscle tendon.

Cathode   Negatively charged electrode.

Cavitation   The vibrational effect on gas bubbles by an ultrasound beam.

Circuit   The path of current from the generating source through the various components back to the generating source.

Coaxial cable   Heavy, well insulated electrical wire where central thick wire component is surrounded by a cylindrical mesh of thin wire.

Collimation   The process of making parallel

Connective tissue   Tissue that supports and connects other tissues and tissue parts.

Contraindications   Special circumstances or symptoms that renders the use of a remedy or procedure inadvisable.

Cryotherapy   Therapeutic use of cold modality.

Diathermy   Therapeutic use of high frequency current to generate the deep heat in the body tissue.

Direct current   An electric current in which there is continuous flow in one direction.

Edema   Localized or generalized excessive collection of tissue fluid

Erythema   Redness of the skin caused by capillary dilation.

Exostosis   Bony outgrowth that arises from the surface of a bone.

Fibroblast   Any cell from which connective tissue is developed.

Fibrosis   Formation of fibrous tissue in the repair process following injury.

Frequency   Number of occurrence of any event per unit time.

Gate control theory   Assumption which states that painful impulses can be prevented from reaching towards the higher levels of central nervous system by stimulation of large sensory nerve fibers.

Hemarthrosis   Blood effusion into a cavity of a joint.

Haematoma   An area of swelling containing clotted blood, which is confined to an organ, tissue or space and caused by a break in blood vessel.

Haemorrhage   Tissue reaction to injury.

Hertz   A unit of frequency equal to one cycle per second.

Insulator   Substance or the body that interrupt the transmission of electricity to surrounding object by conduction.

Indication   The reason to prescribe a remedy or procedure or modality.

Ion   A positively or negatively charged particle.

Laser   Acronym for the light amplification of stimulated emission of radiation. A beam of power can also be termed a Laser.

Marasmus   Form of protein energy malnutrition predominantly due to severe caloric deficit.

Melanin   A group of dark brown or black pigments that occur naturally in the eye, skin, hair and other tissues.

Modulation   Alteration in the parameters of current to prevent accommodation.

Phagocyte   A cell that consumes foreign material and debris.

Photokeratitis   Inflammation of the eyes caused by exposure to ultraviolet rays.

Phonophoresis   Transfer of drug molecules into the tissue by the use of ultrasound.

Piezoelectric effect   Generation of electrical change across the crystal of piezoelectric substance on application of pressure or compression.

Photon   A packet or quantum of light energy.

Plica   Thickened synovial fold.

Psoralen   Photosensitive drug. Methaoxypsoralen, trimethyl-psoralen and other chemicals of similar make-up.

Pulsed ultrasound   Method of administering ultrasound in which the emission of the sound waves is intermittent.

Radiation   Process by which energy is propagated through the space or emission of energy in all directions from a common center.

Reverse piezoelectric effect   Deformation or oscillations of crystal of piezoelectric substance on application of electricity.

Spasm   An involuntary of contraction of muscle that is protective in nature. It can occur in visceral and skeletal muscles.

Spasticity   Increased tone of muscles due to upper motor neuron lesion.

Sprain   An injury of ligament, which is less than complete.

Stimulated emission   When a photon interacts with an atom already in a high energy state and decay of the atomic energy occurs, releasing two photons.

Strain   An injury of muscle, which is less than complete.

Substantia gelatinosa   Gray matter of the spinal cord surrounding the central canal.

Tendonitis   Inflammation of a tendon of muscle.

Thermotherapy   The use of the heat in the treatment of diseases and disorders.

Transducer   A device that changes energy from one form to another.

Trigger point   Any localized area of body that when stimulated by pressure causes a sudden pain in a specific area.

Ultrasound   Inaudible sound waves with a frequency in the range of 20,000 to 10 billion.

Vasoconstricrion   Decrease in the lumen of vessels.

Vasodilation   Increase in the lumen of vessels.

Viscocity   Relative position of fluid particles due to attraction of molecules to each other.

Wavelength   The distance between the beginning and end of a single wave cycle.

References and Suggested Reading

1. Behrens Barbara J, Michlovitz Susan L: Physical Agents, Theory and Practice for the Physical Therapist Assistant, FA Davis company, Philadelphia, 1996.
2. Bonica JJ: The Management of Pain, vol. II Lea, Febiger, Malvem PA, 1990 and I.
3. Dolphin S, Walker M: Healing Accelerated by Ionozone Therapy, Physiotherapy, 1979, 65:81-82.
4. Foster Angela, Palastanga Nigel: Clayton's Electrotherapy; Theory and Practice, AITBS Publishers, New Delhi, 2000, 9th ed.
5. Kahn J: Principles and Practice of Electrotherapy, Churchill Livingstone, New York, 1994, 3rd ed.
6. Khandpur RS: Handbook of Biomedical Instrumentation, Tata McGraw-Hill Publishing Company Ltd., New Delhi, 1987.
7. Kitchen Shcila, Bazin Sarah: Clayton's Electrotherapy, 10th ed, PRSIM Indian edition.
8. Kovacs R: Electrotherapy and Light Therapy, Lea and Febiger, Philadelphia, 1949.
9. Krusen FH, Kotke FJ, Euwood PM: Handbook of Physical Medicine and Rehabilitation, WB Saunders Company, Philadelphia, 1971.
10. Lehman GF, De Lateur BJ: Therapeutic Heat and Cold, Williams and Wilkins, Baltimore, 1982, 3rd ed.
11. Licht S: Electrodiagnosis and Electromyography, Elizabeth Licht, New Haven, 1971, 3rd ed.
12. Low J, Reed Ann: Electrotherapy Explained: Principles and Practice, Butterworth Heinemann, London, 1990.
13. Michloeitz SL: Thermal Agents in Rehabilitation, FA Davis, Philadelphia, 1990.
14. Kuprian W: Physical Therapy for Sports, WB Saunders Company, Philadelphia, 1995, 2nd ed.
15. Prentice WE: Therapeutic Modalities in Sports Medicine, Times mirror Mosby College publishing, St. Louis, 1990.

16. Robinson AJ, Madder LS: Clinical Electrophysiology, Williams and Wilkins, Baltimore, 2nd ed, 1994.
17. Savage B: Interferential Therapy, Faber and Faber, Bostan, 1984.
18. Wadsworth H, Chanmugan APP: Electrophysical Agents in Physiotherapy, Marrickvifle, NSW, Australia, Science Press, 1980.
19. Walsh DM, McAdams ET; TENS: Clinical Applications and Related Theory, Churchill Livingstone, New York, 1997.
20. Wolf SC: Electrotherapy, Churchill Livingstone, New York, 1981.

Index

READER SUGGESTIONS SHEET

Please help us to improve the quality of our publications by completing and returning this sheet to us.

Title/Author: **Basics of Electrotherapy by Subhash Khatri**

Your name and address:

E-mail address,

Phone and Fax:

How did you hear about this book? [please tick appropriate box (es)]

☐ Direct mail from publisher   ☐ Conference   ☐ Bookshop

☐ Book review   ☐ Lecturer recommendation   ☐ Friends

☐ Other (please specify)   ☐ Website

Type of purchase: ☐ Direct purchaseBookshop ☐   Friends ☐

Do you have any brief comments on the book?

Please return this sheet to the name and address given below.

JAYPEE BROTHERS
MEDICAL PUBLISHERS (P) LTD
EMCA House, 23/23B Ansari Road, Daryaganj
New Delhi 110 002, India